Fighting Fat

Break the Dieting Cycle and Get Healthy for Life!

One size does not fit all

Steven Lamm, M.D.

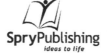

SpryPublishing
ideas to life

This edition is published by Spry Publishing LLC
315 East Eisenhower Parkway, Suite 2
Ann Arbor, MI 48108 USA

Printed and bound in the United States of America.

10 9 8 7 6 5 4 3 2

Library of Congress Control Number: 2014950377
Paperback ISBN: 978-1-938170-56-0
E-book ISBN: 978-1-938170-57-7

To my mother-in-law Yvonne Kovner,
who demonstrated great courage,
compassion, and caring in her life.

Contents

Introduction

Food Behavior and Psychology
Waste Not, Want Not

Redefining Diet
The Diet Paradox
Your Metabolism and Diets
What's My RMR?
Can We Change Our Metabolism?
The Hormone Backlash
Your Doctor's Role, Reframed

Health at Every Size
Fit but Fat
Numbers Beyond the Scale
Healthy Eating and Movement
Fighting the Stereotypes

Medication: A Double-Edged Sword
Drugs That Promote Weight Gain
Are Weight Loss Drugs Right for You?
Today's Weight Loss Drugs
Diabetes Drugs and Weight Loss Benefits
The Future of Weight-Management Drugs

A Physician/Patient Story
What Is Bariatric Surgery?
How It Works
Is It Right for You?
When Bariatric Surgery Isn't Your Best Option
Getting in the Right Frame of Mind
Teamwork

Introduction

Unless you have been living on a desert island or otherwise cut off from civilization, you know that weight problems have reached epidemic proportions in America. Two of every three adults are overweight or obese, driving up healthcare costs and disability and causing dramatic declines in productivity and quality of life. It is the health crisis of our lifetime. And to date, medicine has failed to help those struggling with its fallout.

For nearly a century, the medical establishment has considered obesity a condition of "unsatisfactory dietary bookkeeping," where calories in exceed energy out.[1] This scientific viewpoint is the foundation for the blanket "diet and exercise" prescription doctors still continue to give most patients struggling with weight issues today.[2]

But, what we know about the biology of overweight and obesity has changed dramatically in the past 20 years, and exciting new scientific discoveries are expanding the tool set with which we have to work. Discoveries of key gut hormones and brain pathways that control weight gain and loss have led to new drug and surgical treatments. This is important, because the same body of research explains why, for the majority of people, the traditional prescription of diet and exercise is not enough to achieve significant, sustainable weight loss and related health benefits.

If you've picked up this book, you have probably experienced this firsthand. And, you're looking for a solution to your weight and health issues that actually works. And, you're now wondering why doctors are telling you to "eat less and move more" if it's not a long-term solution for most people. You aren't alone. I wonder why many in the medical profession continue to be satisfied with this advice when it clearly has not been effective. It's obvious we're missing something.

The simple answer is that the new obesity science we explore in this book is still unknown to most doctors who have been in practice for more than five years. But, before you pick up the phone to fire your doctor, understand that there's a reason for this. All physicians learn their basic science and biology in medical school (myself included). Then there are years of hospital training before we start to practice. And, while we have access to new pharmaceutical and treatment options, staying up-to-date on advances in core science concepts requires time and resources most of us don't have. So, we pick and choose our areas of focus, usually those that have the biggest impact on the patients we serve. That's why we have medical specialties; there's simply too much evolving medical science out there for one person to keep up with everything.

And that's okay. As an internist, there are a lot of conditions that I am not up-to-date on, since I am not a specialist that treats them. I am not up-to-date on the latest treatment for psoriasis, or multiple sclerosis, or Parkinson's disease. I don't see patients for these conditions, and if I do, I refer them to the dermatologist, or neurologist, or geriatrician who can provide them with the specialized care they need.

Obesity, however, is a different story. With two-thirds of Americans overweight or obese today, the odds are that every primary care provider in this country has a daily encounter with a patient needing informed guidance on weight-related health problems. To be on the front lines of primary care demands that we become educated in the science of weight management and understand the root of the problem. Internists such as myself, family practice doctors, pediatricians, cardiologists, and other physicians seeing these patients on a regular basis owe it to them to stay current in this field. We can't afford not to.

Recently, the *Journal of the American Medical Association* published an editorial that summed up the problem with traditional approaches to weight management beautifully: "Attempts to lower body weight without addressing the biologic drivers of obesity ... will inevitably fail for most individuals."[3] Now, it's not too often that I agree with editorials, but this one I applaud. Those biologic drivers the authors refer to change the way our metabolism, our hormonal systems, and nervous system wiring works in an adaptive effort to "protect" us against weight loss. The truth is that if you are struggling with excess weight, your body is working against you. We need to stop setting the obese and overweight up for failure by ignoring this fact.

Just as important as staying current in obesity science is that physicians recognize the very individual nature of each person who struggles with weight issues and set more effective goals focused on health, not pounds. Someone who is 100 pounds overweight and dealing with high blood pressure and joint pain can benefit tremendously from taking off just 20 percent of their excess weight versus focusing on the entire 100 pounds. On the other side of the coin, there are also people who are overweight, yet metabolically fit, who may not require any intervention at all.

You, the patient, play the most important role in the battle against obesity-related health. None of the available treatments we have will work without your commitment to real-life changes. Denial is one of the strongest and most protective emotional mechanisms we have; when it prevents us from recognizing the gravity of a weight-related health issue, it can be harmful, even fatal. To manage weight and health, you need to acknowledge the problem and give your doctor permission to help you.

There is still a gap between the new science of obesity and the ability to translate and implement it into actionable treatments that make a clinical impact on weight-related health issues. The holy grail of weight management has not yet been discovered, but I have no doubt that with the way obesity science is progressing, it is coming. The gap is narrowing.

In the meantime, we have a pretty effective arsenal of treatment options that target the biological triggers of weight gain and take the patient's lifestyle and personal needs into consideration. For some, effective treatment is drug therapy, and for others surgery may be the answer. Many struggling with weight can benefit from better sleep hygiene (a variety of different practices that are necessary to have normal, quality nighttime sleep and full daytime alertness) and stress management. And, yes, the composition of the diet and changes in the intensity and the nature of physical activity do make a difference in your overall health and are part of the obesity equation (they just aren't the whole solution for most people).

Wider and more affordable access to nutrient-dense foods is also a barrier to better health that a number of organizations are working to change (the resource section in the back of this book lists some of these programs). Just as important as finding these foods is understanding how to prepare them. I recently had the privilege of meeting David Bouley, a chef and award-winning restaurateur who is passionate about the science of nutrition. He understands food science and how to pick and prepare healthy foods for maximum nutritional ben-

Step-by-Step Plan for Fighting Fat

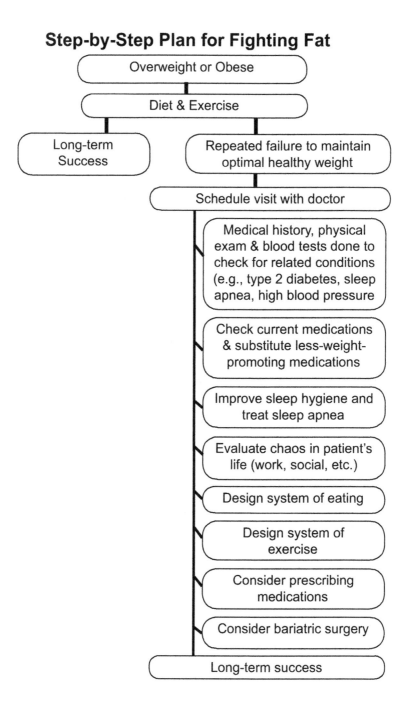

Overweight or Obese

Diet & Exercise

Long-term Success

Repeated failure to maintain optimal healthy weight

Schedule visit with doctor

Medical history, physical exam & blood tests done to check for related conditions (e.g., type 2 diabetes, sleep apnea, high blood pressure

Check current medications & substitute less-weight-promoting medications

Improve sleep hygiene and treat sleep apnea

Evaluate chaos in patient's life (work, social, etc.)

Design system of eating

Design system of exercise

Consider prescribing medications

Consider bariatric surgery

Long-term success

efit. Through educational programs integrating holistic health and nutrition science, Bouley and others like him are sharing those skills with others and changing the way the public and the healthcare profession think about food.

These types of real-world programs are a 180-degree change from the majority of diet books and commercial programs that have, in the past, been the fallback resource for most people struggling to gain health and lose weight. But, eating according to some astrological sign is not helpful advice for treating obesity. It diminishes the seriousness of the disease, and more importantly, it doesn't work long term. This is not a diet book. You'll find no magic fat-burning food formula or prescriptive menu plans here. Instead, it's a road map to help you find your individual path to better health.

The first step on this path is your doctor's office. Bring this book with you to your next appointment. Use the checklists within it to prompt an open conversation about your weight and treatment options. If your doctor is not familiar with the new obesity science, this book is a great introduction for him. Together, you can find a way to work toward the goal of a healthier, happier you—focusing on wellness, not weight.

References

1. What causes obesity? *JAMA*. 1924; 83(13):1003.
2. McLester JS. The principles involved in the treatment of obesity. *JAMA*. 1924; 82(26): 2103–2105. doi:10.1001/jama.1924.02650520009006.
3. Ludwig DS, Friedman MI. Increasing adiposity: Consequence or cause of overeating? *JAMA*. 2014; 311(21): 2167–2168. doi:10.1001/jama.2014.4133.

CHAPTER 1

A National Crisis

David's Story

David is a 41-year-old information technology (IT) executive who is visiting his doctor for an annual physical at the request of his wife. He doesn't want to be there. Since his last visit, two years ago, he has put on 30 more pounds. And, at that time, David's doctor mentioned that he should really be about 20 pounds lighter and told him to "watch what you eat and try to get to the gym more often." But with working long hours at a stressful job, neither of those things happened. David did drop about 20 pounds by going on a protein shake plan a coworker recommended, but six months later he had gained it all back and then some.

David's weight has been an issue all of his adult life, and he's tried just about every book, bar, shake, gadget, and gimmick out there. He knows he needs to lose weight—his doctor has told him to diet and exercise more than once. But, every time he makes some progress, he finds himself even heavier within a year. Now his weight is starting to infringe on his quality of life; he is finding it harder to breathe, his energy is low, his knees hurt, and he is having trouble sleeping. He feels like a failure and isn't sure where to turn.

A National Crisis

The obesity epidemic represents what is arguably the biggest failure in the history of American medicine. More than two-thirds of the adult population is overweight or obese, and 17 percent of our children between the ages of 2 and 19 are obese.[1] Despite a lucrative $60-billion-a-year consumer weight loss industry and several federal initiatives launched in the past decade to attack the obesity problem, we simply aren't making any headway.[2]

Over the past 50 years, obesity rates have steadily climbed (Figure 1). As a leading contributor to high-cost conditions such as heart disease, stroke, and type 2 diabetes, America's weight problem now represents our biggest health expense, estimated at upward of $190 billion annually.[3] A person who is obese can expect to pay $1,500 more in medical costs each year than someone who is not.[4] And, there's a higher price to pay, as one in five deaths in the United States can be linked to obesity. If the trend continues unchecked, for the first time in over a century life-expectancy rates may actually start to decline in the United States.[5]

Who Is at Fault?

Why aren't things improving? The answer is complex, and there's enough blame—or accountability—to go around. Let's start with the medical community that has historically left the challenge of weight loss to the private sector and continues to prescribe "diet and exercise" to patients struggling with weight, despite mounting scientific evidence that this is perpetuating the problem.

Then there's the long-held American attitude of obesity as a character flaw versus a very real biological condition

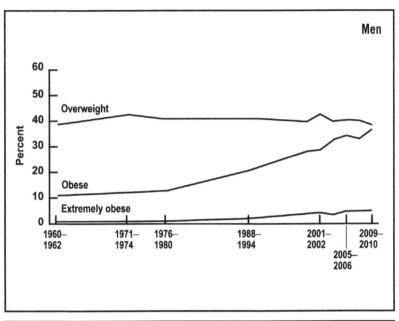

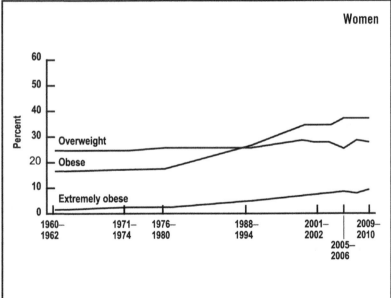

Figure 1. The graphs illustrate the rise of obesity and extreme obesity since 1960.
Sources: CDC/NCHS, National Health Examination Survey.

completely unrelated to willpower. Unfortunately, even some healthcare providers continue to hang on to this bias. That's not to say that the patient has no responsibility, as too often those struggling with weight issues will not go to their physician for help and instead turn to fad diets and self-help books to try and solve the problem.

Finally, our public and private sectors carry responsibility as well. A large proportion of the American food industry drives practices that make unhealthy eating an American's most affordable option. We also have federal government programs that have subsidized and regulated our children out of healthy school lunches and have promoted dietary guidelines that may be contributing to the obesity problem.

So, you now see how our approach to obesity is collectively America's biggest challenge. But, it can also be our biggest opportunity, for if we work together to tackle it across all these sectors, we can not only reduce obesity, but improve all Americans' health and quality of life. We need a very bold new initiative, based on science and clinical experience, to push the needle down on the national scale.

Shifting Our Fat Bias

One significant step toward this goal was taken in 2013, when the American Medical Association announced it would change policy to classify obesity as a chronic disease requiring a range of medical treatments and interventions. The change is expected to prompt insurers to reimburse for a wider range of obesity treatments and to heighten physicians' awareness of the seriousness of obesity.

This policy also reflects our growing knowledge of the biology of obesity and the scientific discoveries we have made over the past 20 years. Our knowledge base and understanding of the biological mechanisms of weight gain are deeper than ever. Researchers are unlocking the secrets of hunger and the sense of fullness (satiety), metabolism, and the complex gut hormones that can help or hinder weight loss, and discovering the different parts of the brain that are involved with the regulation of eating and energy.

All of these advances mean that treatments are beginning to emerge that offer overweight and obese people real options beyond the traditional "diet and exercise" prescription. People struggling with weight problems and accompanying chronic health complications are finally getting some new tools to work with to regain their health. And this is a good thing, because long-term studies show that more than half of overweight and obese people who lose weight through a diet and exercise regimen will regain it all within five years thanks to the physiological changes that occur when we "diet."[6] And only one in six obese Americans who manage to lose weight can sustain just 10 percent of that weight loss for a year.[7]

A Word on "Diet and Exercise"

Despite this substantial fail rate of diet and exercise to sustain significant long-term weight loss, I want to be clear that eating healthy foods and being physically active certainly are of major benefit in promoting wellness for everyone. The quality of the food we eat plays an enormous role in weight management. Mounting research shows that carbohydrate control may be the real key to managing weight for the long haul, and America's fixation on low-fat food products may be fueling our weight gain. And, of course, the myriad benefits of physical activity for our physical and mental health are indisputable.

I would venture to guess that if you're reading this book, you have tried one or more of the commercial miracle diets out there. The "Results are not typical" disclaimer shown in fine print on the "After" photos in diet ads really should be taken to heart. Time after time, with every new diet that emerges, there is some temporary success for a small number of people, but ultimately, it's not sustainable and the weight comes back. What may be setting us up for failure is the widespread perception of "diet and exercise" as an unrealistic, grueling short-term regimen to reach a goal versus a sustained lifestyle change that is enjoyable. In addition, our biology is working against us, as this kind of weight loss can trigger changes to hormonal systems that actually promote weight regain.

Now, diet and exercise obviously do work for some people who manage to keep that weight off for the long haul. The people who succeed with this approach are usually those who avoid short-term popular "diets" and instead pursue healthy eating habits for life. Their success also reinforces the very individual nature of weight control, in that there is no one blanket solution that works for everyone.

One Size Doesn't Fit All

One thing the new science has made clear to those of us in medicine is that when it comes to weight, every person requires an individualized approach. One size truly doesn't fit all. Beyond the number on the scale, a person's age, health history, occupation, social supports, and economic status each play a part in finding a path to weight control and wellness that will work for them.

So, the 40-year-old man who is 75 pounds overweight and who is suffering from a potpourri of medical issues from sleep disorders to type 2 diabetes to sexual problems, whose occupation requires overnight shiftwork, and who has tried—and failed—to keep off the weight at least a dozen times, may need a surgical solution to regain his health.

But, the 40-year-old woman who is 30 pounds overweight, but is physically active and has perfect blood pressure, cholesterol levels, and overall health, may not need any medical intervention at all. And, a 22-year-old patient who is 15 pounds overweight and who has high blood pressure and prediabetes, and who lives alone and relies on fast food for 50 percent of his diet, may benefit from drug therapy.

The key is assessing each person holistically, both to look at how excess weight is affecting their health and quality of life and to find a solution that is realistic for their lifestyle.

Recalibrating the Goal

In 2009, there were nearly 3 million obesity-related hospital admissions.[8] Being overweight is linked to a laundry list of serious chronic health conditions, including heart disease, high blood pressure, type 2 diabetes, osteoarthritis, and certain types of cancer. These conditions that obesity leads to result in greater mortality and a tremendous decrease in quality of life.

The good news is that, with a loss of as little as 5–10 percent of body weight, you can reap huge benefits by improving these health conditions. Moderate weight loss reduces the risk for heart attack and stroke;[9] improves self-esteem;[10] reduces the risk of developing type 2 diabetes;[11] improves long-term blood sugar control (A1C) and blood pressure;[12] lessens pain and improves mobility;[13] reduces liver inflammation and fatty change in the liver;[14] improves fertility;[15] and improves sleep quality for you and your partner resulting in increased energy.[16] Figure 2 illustrates the health benefits of moderate weight loss in the obese.

This is why, as a doctor, I have a new goal for my over-

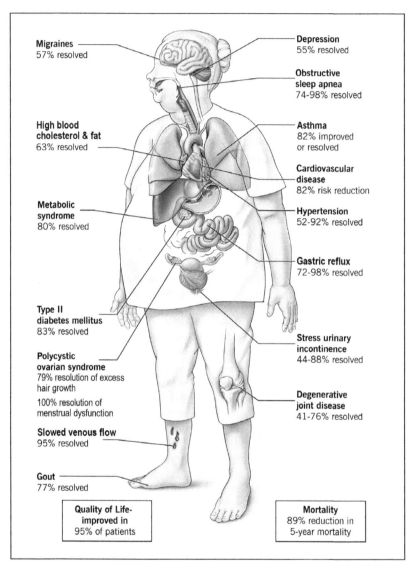

Migraines
57% resolved

High blood
cholesterol & fat
63% resolved

Metabolic
syndrome
80% resolved

Type II
diabetes mellitus
83% resolved

Polycystic
ovarian syndrome
79% resolution of excess
hair growth

100% resolution of
menstrual dysfunction

Slowed venous flow
95% resolved

Gout
77% resolved

Depression
55% resolved

Obstructive
sleep apnea
74-98% resolved

Asthma
82% improved
or resolved

Cardiovascular
disease
82% risk reduction

Hypertension
52-92% resolved

Gastric reflux
72-98% resolved

Stress urinary
incontinence
44-88% resolved

Degenerative
joint disease
41-76% resolved

Quality of Life-
improved in
95% of patients

Mortality
89% reduction in
5-year mortality

Figure 2. The health benefits with a loss of as little as 5–10 percent of body weight. Adapted from the Cleveland Clinic Foundation.

weight patients. It's not to achieve ideal body weight, but instead to reduce these medical complications associated with the weight. We don't yet have the knowledge or the tools to achieve ideal body weight, but we do have the capacity to help patients lose enough weight to lower blood pressure or better control their diabetes.

If I can guide my patients to drop enough weight to reduce the amount of medication they require, and to better manage or even eliminate their medical complications, that's a success story. The bottom line is that it's all about health gained, not weight lost.

A Moonshot Effort

This brings us back to the challenge we are facing—working together to solve the enormous health crisis caused by obesity in this country. And, just as everyone has had a role in the problem, we all play a part in the solution.

What can doctors do? First, they need to ask their patient's permission to discuss weight as a component of health. They can speak to their patients who are overweight at *every* visit. They can make it a real conversation, and not just say "lose weight," and establish goals and provide specific and clear-cut steps for the patient to follow (see chapter 10 for a detailed look at my approach to a meaningful doctor's visit). To do all of this, they need to learn and understand the new science. Fairly recent scientific discoveries such as leptin and ghrelin and neuropeptides (all covered in this book) are things that most doctors probably did not study in medical school.

For their part, patients can give their healthcare providers permission to broach the subject of weight with them. Overweight and obesity are medical issues requiring collaborative treatment. If you have a weight problem, stop trying to fix it all by yourself. Self-help books and packaged food programs are not the answer. If you had cancer or heart disease, you would go to a doctor for help. This is no different.

Friends, family, and coworkers of those struggling with weight problems: you play a role, too. Shed your fat bias. Take the time to read through this book and see the science that proves, unequivocally, that obesity is a disease process that can't be managed through sheer willpower. Those who buy into the myth that excess weight is a character defect make it that much harder for those struggling with weight to seek professional help.

The roles of agriculture, government, and the food industry in stopping obesity are large and complex, and exploring them in depth is outside the scope of this book. But, to bring it back to basics, we need to reward industry for creative solutions that facilitate healthy eating and good nutrition and promote ways to make nutrient-dense food affordable to the masses and widely available everywhere—at the school cafeteria, local ethnic food shops, and in grocery stores across middle America.

Only with this monumental, collective effort, an effort that touches all Americans, will we start to reverse the tide of obesity in this country. Let's start changing things today by working together as doctor and patient.

My Solution

As an internist, I see a wide spectrum of patients with weight problems, from the obese who are suffering from serious related health problems to men and women who are overweight, but metabolically healthy. It's critical that we understand—and respect—the individual needs of each patient and treat them thoughtfully and appropriately. In this book, I'll tell you how I work with my overweight patients to get them on the right path to better health and share questions you should ask your doctor to ensure you are getting the best care available.

This journey should be a collaborative effort—between you, your doctor, and any appropriate specialists. This book is a reflection of that collaborative spirit. I've invited several leading physician specialists to contribute their knowledge of some of the most recent, cutting-edge advances in weight loss treatment. They, too, will explain what options are available for you to discuss with your doctor.

David, Revisited

When David's doctor started to repeat the same old "diet and exercise" refrain at his physical, David pleaded: "Please tell me what diet and exercise you're talking about. Because I think I've tried all of them and I've yet to find the one that actually works." Realizing David's level of frustration, and the less-than-helpful nature of his advice, David's doctor apologized. They spent the next 15 minutes talking about David's past efforts, the obstacles that prevented him from succeeding, and his goals for weight loss and health improvement. David left the appointment with a referral to a registered dietitian who specializes in weight management and the phone number of an exercise physiologist. Most importantly, David was given a follow-up appointment to have a more thorough discussion about the impact his weight was having on his health and life and to create a treatment plan.

References

1. Ogden CL, Carroll MD, Kit BK, Flegal KM. Prevalence of childhood and adult obesity in the United States, 2011–2012. *JAMA*. 2014; 311(8): 806–814. doi:10.1001/jama.2014.732.
2. Marketdata Enterprises. *The U.S. weight loss market: 2014 status report and forecast.* February 2014.
3. Cawley J, Meyerhoefer C. The medical care costs of obesity: An instrumental variables approach. *J Health Econ*. 2012; 31(1): 219–230.
4. Finkelstein EA, Trogdon JG, Cohen JW, Dietz W. Annual medical spending attributable to obesity: Payer- and service-specific estimates. *Health Aff* (Millwood). 2009 Sep–Oct; 28(5): 822–31. doi: 10.1377/hlthaff.28.5.w822. Epub 2009 Jul 27.
5. Masters RK, Reither EN, Powers DA, Yang YC, Burger AE, Link BG. The impact of obesity on US mortality levels: The importance of age and cohort factors in population estimates. *Am J Public Health*. October 2013, 103(10): 1895–1901.
6. Sarwer DB, von Sydow Green A, Vetter ML, Wadden TA. Behavior therapy for obesity: Where are we now? *Curr Opin Endocrinol Diabetes Obes*. 2009 Oct; 16(5): 347–52. doi: 10.1097/MED.0b013e32832f5a79.
7. Blomain ES, Dirhan DA, Valentino MA, Kim GW, Waldman SA. Mechanisms of weight regain following weight loss. *ISRN Obesity*. 2013, Article ID 210524. doi:10.1155/2013/210524.
8. Weiss AJ (Truven Health Analytics), Elixhauser A (AHRQ). Obesity-related hospitalizations, 2004 versus 2009. *HCUP Statistical Brief #137*. July 2012. Agency for Healthcare Research and Quality, Rockville, MD. Available at http://www.hcup-us.ahrq.gov/reports/statbriefs/sb137.pdf.
9. Jensen MD, et al. 2013 AHA/ACC/TOS guideline for the management of overweight and obesity in adults. *Obesity*. 2014;22(S2):S1–S410. Published online before print November 12, 2013.
10. Blaine BE, Rodman J, Newman JM. Weight loss treatment and psychological well-being: A review and meta-analysis. *J Health Psychol*. 2007 Jan; 12(1): 66–82.
11. Merlotti C, Morabito A, Ceriani V, Pontiroli AE. Prevention of type 2 diabetes in obese at-risk subjects: A systematic review and meta-analysis. *Acta Diabetol*. 2014 Oct;51(5):853–63. doi: 10.1007/s00592-014-0624-9. Epub 2014 Aug 2.
12. Henry RR, Chilton R, Garvey WT. New options for the treatment of obesity and type 2 diabetes mellitus (narrative review). *J Diabetes Complications*. 2013 Sep–Oct; 27(5): 508–18.
13. Bliddal H, Leeds AR, Christensen R. Osteoarthritis, obesity and weight loss: Evidence, hypotheses and horizons—a scoping review. *Obes Rev*. 2014 Jul; 15(7): 578–86.

14. Dyson J, Day C. Treatment of non-alcoholic fatty liver disease. *Dig Dis.* 2014; 32(5): 597–604.
15. Sirmans SM, Pate KA. Epidemiology, diagnosis, and management of polycystic ovary syndrome. *Clin Epidemiol.* 2013; Dec 18; 6: 1–13.
16. Jordan AS, McSharry DG, Malhotra A. Adult obstructive sleep apnoea. *Lancet.* 2014 Feb 22; 383(9918): 736–47.

Tips for Talking to Your Doctor

Which of my health problems are directly related to excess weight (if any)?

_____

_____

_____

_____

What's the minimum amount of weight I should lose to start improving one or more of my weight-related health problems?

_____

_____

_____

_____

What is my "action plan" for achieving that goal?
(e.g., Do I need to see a specialist? Are drugs or surgery an option? Should I go to a dietitian?)

_____

_____

_____

_____

CHAPTER 2

Why We Get Fat

Rebecca's Story

Rebecca is a 32-year-old woman who is 5'9" tall and weighs 200 pounds. With a body mass index (BMI) of 29.5 (see chart page 39), she is right on the cusp of obesity. Her mother and father are both overweight, as were her grandparents on her mom's side. She has always struggled with her weight; at her slimmest she was 165 pounds, but that was back in high school.

Six months ago she started working third shift at a hotel and has put on an additional 15 pounds since that time. She's always tired, always hungry, and life has become a cycle of eat, work, and sleep—when she can. Rebecca recognizes that her odd work hours are probably part of the problem, but she's worked overnights before and never felt this bad. She fears she may have a serious health problem due to her constant fatigue and is seeing her doctor to try and get at the root of the problem.

The Big Question

Why are we fat? Why do we remain fat despite our sincere desire and best efforts to be thinner? Why do we regain weight after losing weight? Whoever is able to answer these questions will probably win a Nobel Prize.

There's certainly no doubt that there's a relationship between eating and fatness. So, the real question is: Why do we eat too much? Is it really as much under our control as we have deluded ourselves into believing? Why does the body facilitate weight gain and defend against weight loss despite the obvious potential negative impact? Why do certain individuals who get fat remain metabolically well?

And, how do we explain that intelligent, rational, motivated individuals such as judges, governors, doctors, scientists, and actors, whose professional lives and health depend on optimizing their weight, fail as miserably as those individuals with fewer resources?

We do know that the answer involves a complex biological interaction of hunger, a sense of fullness, and metabolism, dictated by genetic coding and activated by environmental triggers. It goes way beyond "eating less and exercising more" and has little to do with willpower. And, while some environmental factors that fuel weight gain can be managed once we understand them, there is much to weight gain that is outside of our ability to influence.

Genetics

Let's start with what we can't control—our DNA. Since the launch of the Human Genome Project in 1990, science has made tremendous gains in figuring out the genetic factors that influence weight gain.

Researchers have also discovered that there are a few rare forms of obesity associated with mutations or variants in a handful of genes. These same genes are known to play important roles in human hunger, food intake, and energy balance. This is called *monogenic obesity* and accounts for a very small fraction of obesity (fewer than 200 cases are documented in the literature).[1]

Much more relevant is the research that has been done on gene variants associated with raising common obesity risk. For example, one gene variation can cause higher circulating levels of the hunger-regulating hormone *ghrelin*. People who have this variation are constantly hungry, even after eating, and also have a greater interest in eating calorie-dense food. In addition, this gene variation also affects how the brain reacts to ghrelin (discussed later in this chapter). There are two other gene variants known to increase obesity risk.[2, 3, 4]

What do all these genetic discoveries mean to you, in a practical sense? After all, there is no genetic testing for obesity risk, so unless you are in a clinical trial, chances are you'll never know if you have one or more of these genetic variants. But, by shedding light on the complex interplay of hunger, fullness, fat storage, and other biological factors, these new genetic discoveries have allowed us to develop new drugs that target the source of the problem.

Dozens of other gene variants are also being studied for their potential roles in weight gain. But, it's important to note that most cases of obesity are thought to be caused not just by a single obesity risk gene variant, but by a number of genetic markers that interact with myriad environmental triggers to produce a "perfect storm" of weight gain and related health issues. This is good news, as it means that we are not necessarily prisoners of our genes; we can change our lifestyle and influence these environmental factors.

Lifestyle

Today, we can get food virtually anywhere, at almost any time of day or night—where we work, learn, play, and shop. We don't even have to leave our cars for it. And, in our quest for convenience, the food supply has become abundant in highly processed foods that are high in calories and low in nutritional value.

We're also spending much more time sitting, both on the job and at home. Almost half of working adults today are in light-activity jobs (e.g., sitting at a desk) with only 2 in 10 working in high-activity jobs (e.g., construction, farming).[5] We work longer hours behind those desks and spend more time getting to the workplace than we did 40 or 50 years ago. This equates to more time sitting in cars or on public transportation, as only a small percentage of working Americans walk to work or commute by bicycle.[6]

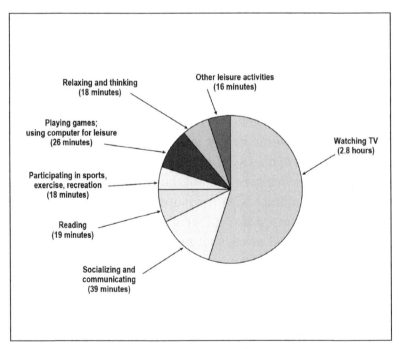

Figure 3. Leisure time on an average day. Total leisure and sports time amounts to roughly 5 hours. *Source*: Bureau of Labor Statistics, American Time Use Survey.

When we do get home, we don't fare much better. On average, Americans aged 15 and older spend a mere 19 minutes a day on sports and other active recreational activities, and the rest is split between television (almost three hours daily) and other passive activities (see Figure 3).[7] For all its benefits, technology has set us back significantly in one respect—the more wired we are, the less physically active our lives become. Three-quarters of American households now have Internet access, and between work and home, we spend more than five hours each day in front of computer and mobile screens consuming digital media.[8] Back in 1984, few of us even had a computer at home.[9]

The big picture is this: Only 52 percent of adult Americans get the recommended 150 minutes or more of weekly exercise needed to be healthy. With roughly half of us not meeting the goal, it's not surprising that two-thirds of America has a weight problem.

Another largely overlooked lifestyle factor that's contributing to our national weight problem is sleep deprivation. Whether we travel extensively, have problems getting to or staying asleep, or have to work nontraditional hours, most of us just don't take enough time recharging our bodies with the recommended 7–9 hours of sleep adults need. And, this lack of sleep causes chaos with the "internal clock" located in our brains and triggered by light signals. This system regulates the production of a number of important hormones, such as melatonin and cortisol. In addition to regulating sleep, these hormones play a large part in metabolism and energy use. When we don't sleep enough, our sensitivity to the sugar-regulating hormone insulin decreases, promoting fat storage. At the same time, levels of the "all full" hormone (leptin) decrease, and the hunger hormone (ghrelin) increase, creating a recipe for weight gain.[10]

Sometimes we don't have a choice in the matter. Almost 15 million Americans work night, evening, rotating, or other irregular schedules.[11] We know that shift work is associated with a host of medical issues, including a higher incidence of metabolic syndrome (a group of risk factors that raises the risk for heart disease and other health problems such as diabetes and stroke), cardiovascular disease, sleep problems, decreased immune function, some cancers, and, of course, obesity.[12] In addition to the lack of sleep they experience, shift workers also don't eat at appropriate times and often don't exercise regularly and consistently, compounding the problem. But, there are steps we can take to help lessen the impact of shift work.

Even if we can theoretically eat better, move more, and get enough sleep, once you start factoring in the reality of life—from work and family demands to economic constraints—the task gets harder. As a doctor, I have to appreciate that people have limitations and work with them to overcome some of those barriers. And, this is where treating each person as an individual is key.

Improving your physical fitness is under your control. While we don't each have an equal ability to become fit, and we all have barriers to overcome, we can all make some progress toward the goal. Park in the back of the lot at work. Take the dog around the block when you get home instead of heading for the couch. Shop for your own groceries instead of having them delivered. There are dozens of small, almost unnoticeable changes you can make in your daily routine, and together they can add up to significant health benefits.

Eating right can be more of a challenge, as access and cost enter the picture. Depending on where you live in America, fresh produce can be difficult to find and, following the laws of supply and demand, fairly expensive. And, as we've already discussed, your hunger mechanism is biologically regulated and beyond your control. But, you can improve the nutritional benefits of your meals by incorporating more whole, unprocessed fruits and vegetables, increasing fiber, decreasing carbohydrates, and choosing lean proteins. Even if you are eating a larger quantity of food (and calories) than is recommended, if the nutritional quality is good, your health outcomes will be better.

Sleep is probably the most difficult lifestyle factor to take control of on your own, especially if a sleep disorder, such as sleep apnea or restless leg syndrome, is part of the problem. You may be working third shift or have two jobs or have family responsibilities that sabotage your sleep efforts.

It's particularly important for you to let your doctor know if you are having trouble getting 7–9 hours of sleep most nights. If your barrier to good sleep is simply not having enough hours in the day (or night) and changing your schedule is not an option, strategic naps or regulating light exposure may help. Eating small, healthy meals on a regular, scheduled basis can also be useful in fighting hunger and the hormonal forces battling against you. If you are a shift worker, a registered dietitian can work with you to shape a meal plan that fits your schedule. Melatonin (a sleep-regulating hormone) supplementation may also be recommended to help regulate the levels of this important hormone in your body.

If you have apnea, a continuous positive airway pressure (CPAP) device that keeps your airway open to regulate breathing during sleep can help. Some sleep medications may also be helpful, although these should always be monitored by a doctor, as some of these drugs can cause more serious sleep issues with long-term use. Meditation and relaxation exercises, adjusting your sleep environment, and making other small changes to your sleep routine can also reap huge benefits.

It's important to remember that beyond weight control, good sleep, nutrition, and physical activity are essential to every aspect of your health. Chapter 11 has more strategies for managing these lifestyle issues.

Wired for Weight Gain

These genetic and lifestyle factors intersect to effectively wire our biology for weight gain. If you are overweight, the biological cards are stacked against you. Normal hunger and fullness signals become impaired as levels of weight-regulating hormones and neurotransmitters (a substance that transmits nerve impulses) are altered, and your body stops responding appropriately to them. As a result, your hunger increases and your energy expenditure, or calorie burn, decreases.

I call this the fat paradox. The fatter a person gets, the easier it is for them to keep getting fatter. Fat cells essentially facilitate more fat. We'll talk more about this in the next chapter when we take a closer look at the fat cell. The size and makeup of our fat (adipose tissue) play a critical part in managing weight gain.

In the past 20 years, researchers have made great strides toward a better understanding of this physiology of weight gain through identification of two key chemicals that regulate our appetite and metabolism.

- *Leptin* is a hormone produced by our fat cells. The hormone sends the "all full" signal to the brain to tell it to reduce hunger and increase energy expenditure. So, you see how leptin can be useful in controlling our weight and helping researchers develop drugs that alter leptin levels and pathways. Unfortunately, studies have shown us that when you lose a large amount of weight, this helpful appetite-regulating hormone actually decreases. This explains why many people always feel hungry after losing large amounts of weight. And, somewhat counterintuitively, research has found that obese people actually have high levels of leptin, but the pathways of the hormone become altered and their body can't use it properly (known as *leptin resistance*).[13]

• **Ghrelin** is produced by the stomach and is often called the "hunger hormone." It has the exact opposite effect of leptin—it tells our brain we are hungry and slows down our metabolism to burn energy and body fat more slowly. And, similarly to leptin, when we lose large amounts of weight, our body fights us to gain it back by increasing ghrelin levels. Scientists have also made the unexpected discovery that obese people produce lower levels of ghrelin; this may somehow be related to a higher sensitivity to ghrelin in the obese, and research continues to better understand this phenomenon.[14] One of the reasons gastric bypass surgery (discussed elsewhere in this book) is so effective is that it permanently alters both the production and pathways of ghrelin.

How Dieting Harms Us

So, you see how the body literally sabotages our best efforts at losing weight in a variety of ways. This is one of the reasons so many people lose weight and then gain even more back.

When people lose large amounts of weight through dieting, they have increased hunger. They have decreased energy expenditure and don't burn as many calories. Changes in leptin and ghrelin production alter the signals that are involved with maintaining weight and metabolism. There are changes in the fat, liver, and muscles that somehow are contributing physiologically to regaining the weight, changes that we don't yet fully understand, but continue to research.

Psychologically, not all weight loss is associated with a good outcome, either. We've found that when people have lost a lot of weight, many remain stressed. They're drained by this effort to keep their weight off, which produces some negative effect on their overall sense of well-being. Initially, they're happy that they managed to lose the weight, but they feel an enormous amount of stress in trying to keep their weight off, which may not be healthy.

The reason they feel this way is because they're struggling to fight their biology, and the part of the brain that's involved with rational decision-making (the cortex) is now fighting the part of the brain that is involved with hunger, metabolism, body temperature, and hormone production (the hypothalamus). The cortex simply can't out think these biological processes, and the hypothalamus almost always wins.

We'll take a closer look at the problems surrounding traditional "dieting" for weight loss in chapter 5.

Whatever Works

It's hard to feel optimistic about managing your weight after learning more about how your body is fighting you every step of the way. But, it's important to recognize three things. First, many of these self-preservation mechanisms your body has developed are related to large drops in weight, and we know that small weight reductions can have large health benefits, and this is the ultimate goal. Second, we are developing new medical treatments and behavior change approaches that can help counteract some of these biological barriers. And, third, everyone is different, and with an individual approach tailored

Knowing Your BMI

BODY MASS INDEX AND RISKS OF OVERWEIGHT

HEIGHT (ft/in) \ WEIGHT (lb)	120	130	140	150	160	170	180	190	200	210	220	230	240	250	260	270	280	290	300	310	320	330
4'5"	30	33	35	38	40	43	45	48	50	53	55	58	60	63	65	68	70	73	75	78	80	83
4'6"	29	31	34	36	39	41	43	46	48	51	53	56	58	60	63	65	68	70	72	75	77	80
4'7"	28	30	33	35	37	40	42	44	47	49	51	54	56	58	61	63	65	68	70	72	75	77
4'8"	27	29	31	34	36	38	40	43	45	47	49	52	54	56	58	61	63	65	67	70	72	74
4'9"	26	28	30	33	35	37	39	41	43	46	48	50	52	54	56	59	61	63	65	67	69	72
4'10"	25	27	29	31	34	36	38	40	42	44	46	48	50	52	54	57	59	61	63	65	67	69
4'11"	24	26	28	30	32	34	36	38	40	43	45	47	49	51	53	55	57	59	61	63	65	67
5'0"	23	25	27	29	31	33	35	37	39	41	43	45	47	49	51	53	55	57	59	61	63	65
5'1"	23	25	27	28	30	32	34	36	38	40	42	44	45	47	49	51	53	55	57	59	61	62
5'2"	22	24	26	27	29	31	33	35	37	38	40	42	44	46	48	49	51	53	55	57	59	60
5'3"	21	23	25	27	28	30	32	34	36	37	39	41	43	44	46	48	50	51	53	55	57	59
5'4"	21	22	24	26	28	29	31	33	34	36	38	40	41	43	45	46	48	50	52	53	55	57
5'5"	20	22	23	25	27	28	30	32	33	35	37	38	40	42	45	47	48	50	52	53	55	55
5'6"	19	21	23	24	26	27	29	31	32	34	36	37	39	40	42	44	45	47	49	50	52	53
5'7"	19	20	22	24	25	27	28	30	31	33	35	36	38	39	41	42	44	46	47	49	50	52
5'8"	18	20	21	23	24	26	27	29	30	32	34	35	37	38	40	41	42	44	46	47	49	50
5'9"	18	19	21	22	24	25	27	28	30	31	33	34	36	37	38	40	41	43	44	46	47	49
5'10"	17	19	20	22	23	24	26	27	29	30	32	33	35	36	37	39	40	42	43	45	46	47
5'11"	17	18	20	21	22	24	25	27	28	29	31	32	34	35	36	38	39	41	42	43	45	46
6'0"	16	18	19	20	22	23	24	26	27	29	30	31	33	34	35	37	38	39	41	42	43	45
6'1"	16	17	19	20	21	22	24	25	26	28	29	30	32	33	34	36	37	38	40	41	42	44
6'2"	15	17	18	19	21	22	23	24	26	27	28	30	31	32	33	35	36	37	39	40	41	42
6'3"	15	16	18	19	20	21	23	24	25	26	28	29	30	31	33	34	35	36	38	39	40	41
6'4"	15	16	17	18	20	21	22	23	24	26	27	28	29	30	32	33	34	35	37	38	39	40
6'5"	14	15	17	18	19	20	21	23	24	25	26	27	29	30	31	32	33	34	36	37	38	39
6'6"	14	15	16	17	19	20	21	22	23	24	25	27	28	29	30	31	32	34	35	36	37	38
6'7"	14	15	16	17	18	19	20	21	23	24	25	26	27	28	29	30	32	33	34	35	36	37
6'8"	13	14	15	17	18	19	20	21	22	23	24	25	26	28	29	30	31	32	33	34	35	36
6'9"	13	14	15	16	17	18	19	20	21	23	24	25	26	27	28	29	30	31	32	33	34	35
6'10"	13	14	15	16	17	18	19	20	21	22	23	24	25	26	27	28	29	30	31	32	34	35

Less risk — More risk

BMI < 25 = Healthy weight
BMI 25–29 = Overweight
BMI ≥ 30 = Obese

$$BMI = \frac{lbs.}{inches^2} \times 704 = \frac{Kg}{m^2} \left(\frac{\text{weight in kilograms}}{\text{height in meters}^2}\right)$$

We keep making references to body mass index (BMI) throughout this book. Using this chart, you may determine your BMI. It is important to understand that you do not have to reach an ideal BMI to realize positive health benefits from weight loss. A reduction of 3–5 percent of your total excess body weight may significantly improve weight-related health conditions.

to your specific needs, you and your doctor can tackle those barriers and find a way to reduce your weight that works for you.

There are many paths to weight management. For some people, diet and exercise do work. And, if you only have 10–20 pounds to lose, that may be a reasonable solution. But, for the overwhelming majority of overweight and obese people, additional medical help is necessary to make the move toward better health.

I'd like you to take a step back and rethink your weight objectives, because the good news is that while we might not reach "ideal BMI" strictly by the numbers, we can influence lifestyle factors enough to achieve a healthier weight. And, health needs to be the end game, because there are overweight people who are cardio-metabolically healthy, or "fat but fit," just as there are people of normal body weight who are unhealthy. So, even if we can't normalize your weight, we have to do everything we can to try to shift you to a healthier state and get to normal cholesterol, blood sugar, and blood pressure levels.

New guidelines developed by the American Heart Association, the American College of Cardiology, and the Obesity Society reflect a step toward this new direction in weight management by promoting a "complications-centric" approach to weight loss.[15] In other words, the goal is not achieving an ideal BMI, but improving those health conditions related to excess weight. These guidelines recognize the fact that a weight loss of as little as 3–5 percent can reap significant health benefits in the form of lower triglycerides (a form of fat found in your blood) and improved long-term blood sugar levels (A1C).

That's why it's so important for people who are overweight to actually go to the doctor so they can determine whether they are in the more metabolically fit or less metabolically fit categories, and together create a real action plan toward wellness. The results of a recent study highlight the importance of the goal of wellness. Metabolically fit may be a myth or not last forever. In an analysis of data tracking adults identified as "healthy obese," researchers found that over the course of 20 years, more than half experienced a decline in their metabolic health as measured by blood pressure, cholesterol levels, blood glucose levels, and insulin resistance.[16] Among the remainder, 10 percent had actually lost weight (to a non-obese level) and remained metabolically healthy.

Rebecca, Revisited

Rebecca's labs all come back within normal range, which are both a relief and a frustration to her. But, her doctor tells her that even if she didn't have a similar reaction at her last third-shift job, it's very likely her current low energy and fatigue are directly related to her work hours and the disruption they are causing to her internal clock.

He also explains that even though her lab tests are normal and she isn't suffering any ill effects from her extra weight now, he's concerned about her future health. They make a follow-up appointment for four months. In the meantime, Rebecca says she's going to step up her efforts to exercise outside of work and look for first- and second-shift opportunities.

References

1. Hu F. Genetic predictors of obesity. In: Hu F, ed. *Obesity Epidemiology*. New York City: Oxford University Press, 2008; 437–460.
2. Loos RJ, Lindgren CM, Li S, et al. Common variants near MC4R are associated with fat mass, weight and risk of obesity. *Nat Genet*. 2008; 40:768–75.
3. Almén MS, Jacobsson JA, Shaik JH, et al. The obesity gene, TMEM18, is of ancient origin, found in majority of neuronal cells in all major brain regions and associated with obesity in severely obese children. *BMC Med Genet*. 2010 Apr 9; 11: 58.

4. Schwenk RW, Vogel H, Schürmann A. Genetic and epigenetic control of metabolic health. *Mol Metab.* 1 November 2013; 2(4): 337–347. doi: 10.1016/j.molmet.2013.09.002).

5. Owen N, Sparling PB, Healy GN, Dunstan DW, Matthews CE. Sedentary behavior: Emerging evidence for a new health risk. *Mayo Clin Proc.* 2010 Dec; 85(12): 1138–41.

6. McKenzie B. Modes less traveled: Commuting by bicycle and walking in the United States. 2008–2012, American Community Survey Reports, ACS-26, U.S. Census Bureau, Washington, DC, 2014.

7. Bureau of Labor Statistics. *American Time Use Survey.* 2012.

8. eMarketer. Media consumption among US adults. http://www.emarketer.com/Article/Digital-Set-Surpass-TV-Time-Spent-with-US-Media/1010096. Accessed June 25, 2014.

9. U.S. Census Bureau. *Computer and Internet Access in the United States: 2012.*

10. Copinschi G, Leproult R, Spiegel K. The important role of sleep in metabolism. *Front Horm Res.* 2014; 42: 59–72.

11. Bureau of Labor Statistics. *May 2004 Current Population Survey.* Special Supplement: Workers on Flexible and Shift Schedules.

12. Herichova I. Changes of physiological functions induced by shift work. *Endocr Regul.* 2013 Jul; 47(3): 159–70.

13. Attie AD, Scherer PE. Adipocyte metabolism and obesity. *J Lipid Res.* 2009 Apr; 50 Suppl: S395–9.

14. Zhang N, Yuan C, Li Z, et al. Meta-analysis of the relationship between obestatin and ghrelin levels and the ghrelin/obestatin ratio with respect to obesity. *Am J Med Sci.* 2011 Jan; 341(1): 48–55.

15. Jensen MD, et al. 2013 AHA/ACC/TOS guideline for the management of overweight and obesity in adults. *Obesity* 2013; DOI: 10.1002/oby.20660.

16. Bell JA, et al. The natural course of healthy obesity over 20 years. *J Am Coll Cardiol.* 2015; 65:101–9.

Tips for Talking to Your Doctor

(Choose those that apply to you.)

I sleep _____ hours, on average, most nights.

I don't get enough sleep because:

1. _____

2. _____

3. _____

How can I get a better and longer night's sleep?

_____

_____

_____

I work evening and/or night shifts. What and when should I eat to be healthy? Can you refer me to a registered dietitian to work on a meal plan?

_____

_____

_____

I don't get enough exercise because:

1. _____

2. _____

3. _____

Let's talk about what I might be able to do to change that.

_____

_____

CHAPTER 3

Anatomy of a Fat Cell

Jason's Story

Jason is a 45-year-old man who has been overweight all of his life. He's had some past successes losing (and regaining) 10 to 15 pounds through Weight Watchers®, but with his current BMI at 35, it seems like a drop in the bucket. Jason has had high blood pressure and type 2 diabetes since his mid-30s. He recently has had problems keeping his blood sugar under 300 most days with the oral medication he is on. His A1C is 12.5 percent, significantly higher than his 7 percent goal.

Jason knows that, over time, an elevated A1C level can cause a host of complications from vision and limb loss to kidney disease, so he's here to find out if he should be taking insulin to gain control over his diabetes. He also knows that the excess fat he's been carrying around is slowly draining away his health, energy, and quality of life.

The Fat Organ

Most of us learned in biology class that your skin is the largest organ in your body, covering an area of about 20 square feet on the average adult. But, in the past several decades, science has discovered that skin may actually be number two in the organ lineup. We now know that body fat is much more than just a storage vault for our excess calories. Our fat actually functions as a glandular organ, releasing more than 50 substances—known as *adipokines*—that are linked to a variety of biological processes, including hunger, inflammation, blood pressure regulation, clotting of the blood, and a whole range of metabolic processes involved in the body's normal functioning that impact every aspect of humans' biology and physiology.[1] Given that American men and women average in at 28 and 40 percent body fat, respectively, fat makes the jump to the biggest organ for a large majority of the U.S. population.[2]

The fat organ system is vital for energy storage and survival, but at the same time, you will see that it can also be terribly dangerous to our bodies. It's a careful balance we must understand and strike to stay healthy.

The Fat Cell, Deconstructed

A fat cell (adipocyte) is fairly simple in construction (Figure 4). It has a nucleus, mitochondria, cytoplasm, and other basic organelles (or cell components), surrounded by a thin membrane. But, the fat cell is unique in that it changes size to accommodate its largest element—a semi-liquid cholesterol and triglyceride droplet that makes up most of the cell. The cell can expand to allow for more fat storage when we take in more caloric energy than our body can burn. In adults, fat cells tend to expand rather than reproduce when excess fat is stored in the body. So, most of the time, fat cells get larger rather than multiply.

However, research has now found that there's an exception to this rule. In a 2010 study of adult men and women who were overfed a high-calorie diet for eight weeks, researchers discovered that a gain of as little as 2.6 pounds resulted in the

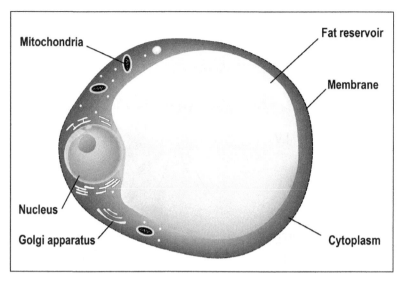

Figure 4. Anatomy of a fat cell (adipocyte, also known as lipocyte).

generation of 2.6 billion new fat cells, shattering a long-held belief that new fat cells stop reproducing after age 20. And, interestingly, all of these new fat deposits were only in the lower body (e.g., hips, thighs, legs). In the upper body, the fat cells merely enlarged.[3]

White Fat and Brown Fat

Most of the fat found in the adult body is made up of white adipocytes, described previously. However, our bodies do contain a small amount of what is called *brown fat*, or *brown adipose tissue* (BAT). Infants and small children have much of this brown fat. It allows them to generate heat in order to maintain their body temperature. As we age, much of this brown fat is converted to white fat. However, we do hang on to some BAT, primarily around organs and in the neck, back, and chest.[4]

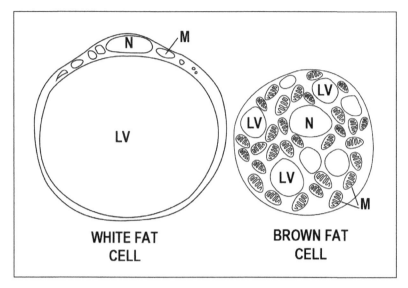

Figure 5. White fat cell (left) and brown fat cell (right). Note the single large lipid vacuole (LV) in the white fat cell and the numerous smaller lipid vacuoles in the brown fat cell. M = mitochondria; N = nucleus.

Brown fat cells are different from white fat in several important ways (Figure 5). Instead of containing one large globule of fat, a brown adipocyte has a number of fat globules distributed throughout. It also contains numerous mitochondria throughout the cell, and this is what gives it a brown color. The mitochondria hold the key to the special role brown fat plays in the body. When activated, the mitochondria in brown fat actually burn the fat within the cell to generate heat and energy. At the same time, they increase uptake of sugar (glucose) from the bloodstream. This means that brown fat can actually burn fat and calories, and even help lower blood sugar levels. All of these are, of course, desirable traits for those of us interested in weight management and diabetes control.[5]

So, what activates the mitochondria furnace in brown fat? One thing is cold. In response to cold temperatures, our body tries to regulate our internal thermostat by burning off this energy. This is why infants are born with little white fat tissue; they have more brown fat than we do as adults to serve this purpose.

The other, more interesting activator of brown fat is a combination of hormones and nerve pathways. We have discovered that certain hormones can set off this fat- and sugar-burning response. This is really the key to some exciting new drug and treatment options in the coming years. Research shows us that people who are obese and those with diabetes actually have less active brown fat cells that are smaller in size than people of normal BMI without diabetes. So, if we can develop a pill that stimulates our brown fat to work overtime, it could be very beneficial to people struggling with diabetes and other obesity-related health issues.

Also promising is the recent discovery that there appears to be a third type of fat cell located along our spine and collarbone, called *beige fat*. Similar to brown fat, beige fat also has numerous mitochondria that burn sugar and fat. While its calorie-burning potential is not as high as that of brown fat, beige fat may also represent another opportunity for new treatment targets as researchers learn more about how it works and what activates it.[6]

Fat Storage and Distribution

Traditionally, we've always thought of fat as our primary storage vault for the body's excess energy. This has served humankind well in times of drought and deprivation, when we needed those fat stores to get us through leaner times. But, in modern society, we are more likely to fill up our fat energy vaults with fuel we'll never burn.

Our fat tissue is both just under the skin (*subcutaneous*)

and around the organs (*visceral*). While we may not like the look of it, subcutaneous fat, the kind that you can grab with your hand, is relatively benign, health wise. It's the deeper fat around the organs that can cause problems.

Most of the fat we accumulate in our lower bodies is just under the skin. Excess amounts of abdominal fat, however, are a combination of subcutaneous fat and deeper visceral fat. You may have heard that an "apple shaped" physique puts you at risk for diabetes and heart disease? This is because of all that visceral fat. Large amounts of visceral fat pump out inflammatory chemicals known as cytokines that can cause a condition in which the body produces insulin but does not use it effectively (insulin resistance), heart disease, and a host of other health problems.

How do you know if you have too much visceral fat? Keep an eye on your waistline. Women with a waist circumference of 35 inches or more and men with a waist circumference of 40 inches or more have a higher risk of cardio-metabolic health problems.

Healthy Fat/Angry Fat

So, as we've seen, fat cells are both friend and foe. With a healthy amount of fat, we have energy reserves, the ability to regulate our temperature, and can even use certain types of fat (i.e., brown and beige) to our metabolic advantage. Think of healthy fat as a cuddly teddy bear that keeps us safe and warm.

But, fat can and does turn on us. When provoked—by stretching our fat cells to their literal breaking point— the cuddly teddy bear becomes a vicious grizzly. Aptly named *angry fat*, our stressed fat tissue unleashes its fury by setting off an immune response that promotes inflammation, insulin resistance, and a multitude of other unwanted side effects.

When these angry fat cells become overstressed and die, two things happen. First of all, white blood cells (macrophages) come in to clean up the mess. A *macrophage* consumes foreign material and dead cells, protecting our body against infection and other dangers. As macrophages perform this clean-up duty, they also trigger the release of cytokines that promote inflammation. This inflammation appears to be one of the more destructive forces contributing not only to arthritis pain, but heart disease, diabetes, and a host of other health issues.

Secondly, when angry fat cells explode, the amount of free fatty acids circulating in the blood goes up, which also contributes to this toxic, pro-inflammatory environment. All of this can have a very detrimental effect on our blood vessels, muscles, heart, liver, pancreas, and brain.

- *Blood vessels.* Fat cells surrounding the coronary arteries are thought to play a central role in the inflammation of blood vessels that triggers buildup of plaque in those vessels (atherosclerosis).[7]
- *Skeletal muscles.* Inflammatory cytokines promote insulin resistance in muscles, so the body is unable to use insulin to effectively process blood glucose for energy.[8]
- *Heart.* Like the skeletal muscles, the muscle of the heart also becomes insulin resistant.[9]
- *Pancreas.* Free fatty acids target the insulin-producing beta cells in the pancreas and damage them.
- *Liver.* Excess fat accumulations on the liver can cause scarring and liver failure.
- *Brain.* Obesity increases the risk of Alzheimer's disease.[10] Early research suggests that cytokines can cross the blood-brain barrier and affect learning and memory.[11]

Fat's Signaling System

So, when we talk about fat as an endocrine organ, this is because of its ability to secrete a variety of chemicals called adipokines. These are a collection of hormones and cytokines (also known as cell-signaling proteins). While it's beyond the scope of this book to explore the role of every adipokine, there are a few key players worth noting.

- *Leptin.* The first of these adipokines, the hormone leptin, was discovered in 1994 and opened the door on the new fat science.[12] Leptin helps regulate appetite and energy use by sending our brains the "all full" signal. When we lose fat mass, leptin levels go down, stimulating appetite to regain what has been lost. And, when we gain fat, leptin increases in order to discourage further weight gain.

  Leptin can work against us, though. Overweight people who lose a significant amount of weight start to feel constantly hungry as their leptin levels compensate. And, overweight and obese people frequently become leptin resistant, and as such, they don't reap the benefits of leptin's natural appetite suppression.

- *Adiponectin.* The other useful adipokine is a substance known as adiponectin. Adiponectin helps regulate sugar levels by increasing insulin sensitivity and breaks down free fatty acids.[13] It may also have some important anti-inflammatory properties, making it potentially helpful in protecting the heart and blood vessels. Unlike leptin, adiponectin levels decrease as body weight rises. So, the people who need it the most—the overweight and obese—tend to have very low levels of this important substance.

We've only scratched the surface of this complex signaling system that is mediated through our fat cells, but the progress we've made has helped us understand the biological link between certain kinds of fat and cardiovascular, immune, and metabolic health problems. That, in turn, is leading the way to new drugs and treatments for weight-related health issues.

Jason, Revisited

Because insulin can cause weight gain, Jason's doctor wants to consider other options. It's clear from Jason's past history that he's made a real effort to lose weight through calorie restriction a number of times over the years, always unsuccessfully. It's also clear he's going to need some additional help bringing down his weight.

Given Jason's high BMI, uncontrolled diabetes, and high blood pressure (hypertension), his doctor thinks he's a perfect candidate for bariatric surgery. He tells Jason about recent research that shows that diabetes symptoms often go into complete remission and blood sugars normalize after certain types of metabolic surgery. Jason seems eager to find a permanent solution to his health problems and willing to make the lifestyle changes required. His doctor refers him to a surgeon. In the meantime, he adds the drug Victoza® (liraglutide) to Jason's oral medication to see if they can bring his blood sugar down without adding insulin to the equation yet.

References

1. Berggren JR, Hulver MW, Houmard JA. Fat as an endocrine organ: Influence of exercise. *J Appl Physiol* (1985). 2005 Aug; 99(2): 757–64. Review. PubMed PMID: 16020439.
2. St-Onge MP. Are normal-weight Americans over-fat? *Obesity* (Silver Spring). 2010 Nov; 18(11): 2067–8. doi: 10.1038/oby.2010.103.

3. Tchoukalova YD, Votruba SB, Tchkonia T, et al. Regional differences in cellular mechanisms of adipose tissue gain with overfeeding. *Proc Natl Acad Sci USA*. 2010 Oct 19; 107(42): 18226–31. doi: 10.1073/pnas.1005259107. Epub 2010 Oct 4.

4. Enerbäck, S. Human brown adipose tissue. *Cell Metab*. 2010 Apr; 11(4): 248–252, ISSN 1550-4131, http://dx.doi.org/10.1016/j.cmet.2010.03.008. (http://www.sciencedirect.com/science/article/pii/S1550413111000078).

5. Sacks H, Symonds ME. Anatomical locations of human brown adipose tissue: Functional relevance and implications in obesity and type 2 diabetes. *Diabetes*. 2013 Jun; 62(6): 1783–90. doi: 10.2337/db12-1430.

6. Wu J, Boström P, Sparks LM, et al. Beige adipocytes are a distinct type of thermogenic fat cell in mouse and human. *Cell*. 2012 Jul 20; 150(2): 366–76. doi: 10.1016/j.cell.2012.05.016. Epub 2012 Jul 12.

7. Stoll LL, Romig-Martin S, Harrelson AL, et al. Isolation and characterization of human epicardial adipocytes: Potential role in vascular inflammation. Program and abstracts from *Experimental Biology* 2006, April 1–5; 2006, San Francisco, California. Abstract 678.2.

8. Wieser V, Moschen AR, Tilg H. Inflammation, cytokines and insulin resistance: A clinical perspective. *Arch Immunol Ther Exp* (Warsz). 2013 Apr; 61(2): 119–25. doi: 10.1007/s00005-012-0210-1. Epub 2013 Jan 10. Review.

9. McGavock JM, Victor RG, Unger RH, Szczepaniak LS; American College of Physicians and the American Physiological Society. Adiposity of the heart, revisited. *Ann Intern Med*. 2006 Apr 4; 144(7): 517–24. Review.

10. Profenno LA, Porsteinsson AP, Faraone SV. Meta-analysis of Alzheimer's disease risk with obesity, diabetes, and related disorders. *Biol Psychiatry*. 2010 Mar 15; 67(6): 505–12. doi: 10.1016/j.bio psych.2009.02.013. Epub 2009 Apr 9.

11. Letra L, Santana I, Seiça R. Obesity as a risk factor for Alzheimer's disease: The role of adipocytokines. *Metab Brain Dis*. 2014 Feb 20. [Epub ahead of print].

12. Zhang Y, Proenca R, Maffei M, et al. Positional cloning of the mouse obese gene and its human homologue. *Nature*. 1994 Dec 1; 372(6505): 425–32. Erratum in: *Nature* 1995 Mar 30; 374(6521):479.

13. Chandran M, Phillips SA, Ciaraldi T, Henry RR. Adiponectin: More than just another fat cell hormone? *Diabetes Care*. 2003 Aug; 26(8): 2442–50. Review.

Tips for Talking to Your Doctor

What's my waist circumference? Do I have too much visceral fat?

CHAPTER 4

The Brain's Role in Obesity

A Word from Dr. Lamm

Norman Sussman, MD, is a psychiatrist who is director of the treatment-resistant depression program at the NYU School of Medicine, and also a colleague of mine at NYU Langone Medical Center (NYULMC). As an expert in the treatment of depression and someone who understands the complex relationship between obesity and mental illness, Dr. Sussman offers a unique perspective on the neurological and psychological aspects of weight and related health issues. I've invited him to share his expertise on the brain's role in obesity here.

Obesity: A Psychological Profile

Obesity has somewhat of a "chicken and egg" relationship with mental health problems. We know that obesity raises the risk of developing mental illness, and we also know that having any mental illness more than doubles a person's chances of being obese.[1]

People who are obese are more likely to have chronic medical conditions and mobility problems that can affect their quality of life and lead to great psychological stress and depression. They are often subjected to weight bias from others that can lead to low self-esteem, another negative influence on mood. Lastly, they are more likely to diet cyclically and have episodes of binge eating, both behaviors that are linked to depression.[2]

In addition, the mentally ill are often propelled toward obesity through the use of antipsychotic and antidepressant drugs that cause weight gain as an unwanted side effect. These drugs affect a number of biological systems that regulate metabolism (the process by which your body converts what you eat and drink into energy) and the sense of fullness. These patients may also use food as a coping and comfort strategy and have poor social supports and increased stress—all of which can lead to obesity.[3]

We do know that depression, in particular, has this inter-dependent relationship with weight gain and obesity. People who are obese have a 55 percent increased risk of developing depression, and depressed people have a 58 percent increased risk of becoming obese.[4] And, obesity and depression feed on each other, magnifying both conditions.

Depression and Weight Gain

Part of the depression-obesity connection can be explained by the neglect of otherwise healthy food choices (apathy) and decreased exercise and physical activity. Depression may fuel a craving for "comfort foods" rich in fats, sugar, and salt—foods that actually may serve as a short-term fix for mood but worsen obesity and related health conditions in the long run.[5]

People with a history of being overweight, and who have successfully achieved weight loss through diet, may become discouraged when they get depressed, losing motivation if they gain just a few pounds. Feeling that it is pointless to keep on trying, they give in and their weight balloons.

Depressed people tend to have a higher BMI, are more likely to smoke cigarettes, and are less likely to be physically active than those without a history of depression. They also are more likely to be single, and this lack of a support network can cause further neglect of their mental and physical health. We know that depression often deters a person from caring for weight-related medical problems such as high blood pressure and diabetes and may prevent a person from taking medication as prescribed.

Clinically, depression can cause weight loss (through loss of appetite) or weight gain (through bingeing, primarily on carbohydrates). The latter type of depression is also associated with oversleeping. People with winter depression—called seasonal affective disorder (SAD)—also start to sleep excessively and crave carbohydrates in the fall and winter months. Some regard this as an underlying form of hibernation traits from earlier in human evolution.

Many, if not most, drugs used to treat depression can cause dramatic weight gain. Chapter 7 of this book has more information on drugs that cause weight gain.

Brain Sabotage

While several parts of the brain are hooked into the circuitry that regulates hunger and the sense of fullness, the hypothalamus acts as the main control center. It adjusts food intake via signaling hormones such as leptin, ghrelin, insulin, and neuropeptide Y (NPY). As we discussed earlier, a growing body of research explains how the brain works against obese people to perpetuate the cycle of weight gain and all its related health issues.

Also playing a role in this "brain sabotage" is dopamine, the brain chemical that helps to regulate the body's reward and

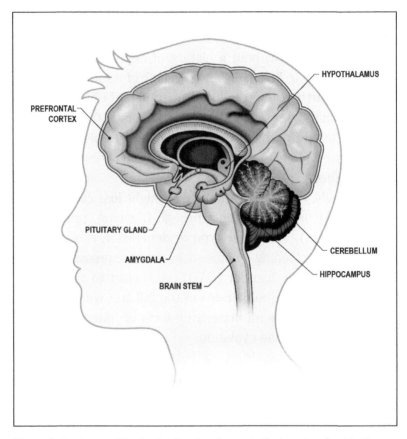

Figure 6. Anatomy of the brain showing the parts that are involved in the hunger/fullness cycle.

motivation system. Dopamine makes us feel good and motivates us toward action. In the obese, the dopamine response system is dampened. The result is that the obese tend to have to eat more than their "normal weight" counterparts to get the same kind of pleasurable response.[6]

We know the hippocampus, the brain region involved with memory, also plays a role in eating behaviors. As one might expect, the hippocampus is associated with food cravings; recalling the taste, smell, or sight of a favorite food can set off a cascade of physiological cues that drive us toward satisfying a craving.[7] We also know that in the obese, the hippocampus becomes hyperactivated in response to food (something that doesn't happen in lean individuals).[8]

How Obesity Impacts Brain Health

Neuroscientists have discovered some fascinating changes in the brain itself that appear to be caused by long-term obesity. When mice are fed high-fat diets to the point of obesity, they experience damage to the circuitry in the hypothalamus. Since we know mice and men are two very different things, the researchers also looked at magnetic resonance imaging (MRI) of the brains of obese humans, where they found a similar injury to the hypothalamus.[9] While further studies are needed to confirm the findings, it appears that this damage may also have an impact on the "feeding signals" that the hypothalamus mediates, resulting in a vicious cycle of overeating and chronic obesity.

Recent animal studies have demonstrated that obesity also weakens the blood-brain barrier, the protective layer that shields the brain from harmful substances, among other functions.[10] Obesity sets off a cascade of systemic inflammation. As a result, circulating free fatty acids and cytokines (inflammatory chemicals produced by visceral fat) cross this weakened blood-brain barrier and trigger hypothalamic inflammation, which has been linked to cognitive decline and dementia. It is also thought that this may be the mechanism that causes the obesity-related brain injuries described above.

Food Behavior and Psychology

There are environmental perceptions that influence how much

and what type of food we eat. They can be as subtle as the size of our plates and as black and white as the information on our food labels. Following are a few of the pitfalls that can change our eating behaviors and lead to added weight gain.

- **Nutrition labels.** Snack foods labeled with a low-fat nutrition claim are more likely to lead to overeating in two ways. First, people tend to feel less guilty about consuming these foods. Secondly, they have an inaccurate perception of the appropriate serving size of these foods.[11]

- **Serving size.** Consumer knowledge of serving (or portion) sizes varies by as much as 20 percent from an actual serving.[12]

- **Calorie underestimation.** People of all sizes tend to underestimate the number of calories in a meal as portion sizes increase.[13] Many people who read the nutritional content on a food label are stunned to realize how small a serving size really is. A food that claims to be only 60 calories per serving may barely satisfy most people's hunger.

- **Packaging.** Super-sized food packaging, such as the kind you can buy at warehouse stores, encourages larger portions by setting a distorted perception of what is "normal."

- **Plate size.** Simply put, if you use bigger plates (or are given bigger plates in a restaurant), you'll eat larger portions and more calories.[14] The same goes for serving bowls.

- **Atmosphere.** Yes, even the lighting, smells, and sounds around you when you eat can influence how much you consume. Soft music can encourage slower eating patterns. Distractions such as television and movies can trigger increased food intake past the point of fullness (sometimes called *mindless* or *distracted eating*).[15] Remember that eating should be seen as a dining experience, where the focus is on the flavors, textures, and even the ambiance of the dining space.

Developing an awareness of these environmental pitfalls and how our minds perceive them is important, as we can avoid many of them with some fairly easy tactics. First, evaluate your kitchen and dining environment to promote appropriate portion sizes. Meal plates should be no bigger than nine inches across. Use smaller or shallower bowls and dishes for serving, and replace short, wide glasses with tall, narrow ones. And, when you sit down for a meal or snack, make food the focus and avoid distractions such as television.

If you are buying super-sized packages of food, take a hard look at the nutritional quality of the food. If it's nutrient poor and calorie rich, it's time to switch to smaller packages (if you must keep it on the shopping list at all). If the food has nutritional value and you buy it in quantity for the economic value, then repackage it in several smaller storage containers when you get home to avoid large portion pitfalls. Extras can be stored in the freezer or on a high shelf in the pantry to discourage quick consumption.

A good dietitian can help educate you on these strategies, as well as teach you how to read nutrition labels, evaluate serving sizes, and plan your meals at an appropriate caloric intake.

Waste Not, Want Not

If your mother always made you clean your plate before you could leave the dinner table, you may already be at a disadvantage when it comes to healthy eating. Many people eat past the point of hunger simply because there is still food on their plates, and they have a psychological barrier with the financial and social implications of throwing away "perfectly good food." This can be particularly true in restaurants where portions are notorious for being large enough for two people.

It's understandable (and commendable) to want to avoid wasting food. But, there are other ways to prevent waste without consuming more calories. These may include splitting your entree with another diner, ordering a la carte, or asking the waiter to box up half of your meal before it comes out of the kitchen so that you can take it home for lunch or dinner the following day.

At home, paying close attention to the portion sizes you dish up is also important. And that's not just for you, but for your children as well. One pitfall of parenthood is the "picking off" of leftover food from a child's plate. Many men and women are already at risk of gaining weight after having children due to hormonal changes, aging, and less parental focus on their own health and appearance. This can be compounded when mom or dad feel that they must eat the fries, chicken nuggets, or burger their child doesn't finish.

Try to focus on your own meals and avoid this picking problem. You should also do your child a favor by getting them on the path to healthy eating from the start. Avoid the traditional kid's menu fare of fast food, and give children reasonable, child-sized portions of nutritious foods so that you can both feel good about a clean plate.

References

1. McElroy SL. Obesity in patients with severe mental illness: Overview and management. *J Clin Psychiatry.* 2009; 70 Suppl 3: 12–21.
2. Mental health and chronic physical illnesses: The need for continued and integrated care. World Federation for Mental Health, 2010.
3. Markowitz S, Friedman MA, Arent SM. Understanding the relation between obesity and depression: Causal mechanisms and implications for treatment. *Clin Psychol: Sci Prac* 2008; 15(1): 1–20.
4. Markowitz S, Friedman MA, Arent SM. Understanding the relation between obesity and depression: Causal mechanisms and implications for treatment. *Clin Psychol: Sci Prac* 2008; 15(1): 1–20.
5. Weltens N, Zhao D, Van Oudenhove L. Where is the comfort in comfort foods? Mechanisms linking fat signaling, reward, and emotion. *Neurogastroenterol Motil.* 2014 Mar; 26(3): 303–15.
6. Volkow ND, Wang GJ, Baler RD. Reward, dopamine and the control of food intake: Implications for obesity. *Trends Cogn Sci.* 2011 Jan; 15(1): 37–46.
7. Haase L, et al. Cortical activation in response to pure taste stimuli during the physiological states of hunger and satiety. *Neuroimage.* 2009; 44: 1008–1021.
8. Bragulat V, et al. Food-related odor probes of brain reward circuits during hunger: A pilot FMRI study. *Obesity.* 2010; 18: 1566–1571.
9. Thaler JP, Yi CX, Schur EA, et al. Obesity is associated with hypothalamic injury in rodents and humans. *J Clin Invest.* 2012 Jan 3; 122(1): 153–62. doi: 10.1172/JCI59660.
10. Arnoldussen IA, Kiliaan AJ, Gustafson DR. Obesity and dementia: Adipokines interact with the brain. *Eur Neuropsychopharmacol.* 2014 Mar 20. pii: S0924-977X(14)00087-X. doi: 10.1016/j.euroneuro.2014.03.002. [Epub ahead of print].
11. Wansink B, Chandon P. Can "low fat" nutrition labels lead to obesity? *Journal of Marketing Research,* 2006, 43: 4 (November): 605–17.
12. Wansink B. Environmental factors that increase the food intake and consumption volume of unknowing consumers. *Annu Rev Nutr.* 2004; 24: 455–79.
13. Wansink B, Chandon P. Meal size, not body size, explains errors in estimating the calorie content of meals. *Ann Intern Med.* 2006; 145(5): 326–32.
14. Wansink B, van Ittersum K. Portion size me: Plate-size induced consumption norms and win-win solutions for reducing food intake and waste. *J Exp Psychol Appl.* 2013 Dec; 19(4): 320–32..
15. Wansink B. Environmental factors that increase the food intake and consumption volume of unknowing consumers. *Annu Rev Nutr.* 2004; 24: 455–79. Review.

Tips for Talking to Your Doctor

Can you evaluate me for depression or refer me to someone who can?

_____

_____

_____

_____

Can any of the psychiatric drugs I'm taking be causing weight gain?

_____

_____

_____

_____

Can you refer me to a registered dietitian or a nutrition class that can educate me on concepts such as nutrition label reading, serving sizes, and meal planning?

_____

_____

_____

_____

Why "Diets" Don't Work

Redefining Diet

Diet comes from the Greek word *diaita*, which means "way of living."[1] And this is the approach that can contribute to improved health—treating diet as an ongoing way of feeding your body with the highest levels of nutrients and a proper balance of fats, carbohydrates, and protein. We need to abandon the concept of "diets" as a short-term, restrictive weight loss tool. As you'll see in this chapter, extreme calorie reduction actually works against our weight loss efforts by slowing our metabolism and pushing the brain/gut axis into defense mode. And, the more faddish and restrictive the diets are, the less likely they are to achieve long-term, sustained weight loss.

The Diet Paradox

An alien visiting our planet to observe American eating habits would probably conclude that dieting (in the non-Greek sense) causes obesity, because the only people who seem to be overweight are those who are continuing to jump from one popular diet trend to another. They wouldn't be too far off. With two-thirds of the adult population currently overweight or obese and the majority of those reporting that they are actively engaged in "dieting" efforts, it's pretty clear that something isn't working here.

We have a growing society of overweight individuals who really *want* to lose weight and have tried repeatedly to do so. An estimated 50–70 percent of obese Americans are actively engaged in weight loss efforts of some kind.[2] Most have followed a variety of commercial diet programs that have been promoted as the answer to their problems, and yet even with best efforts to follow them and drop the pounds, they have not been successful for the long term. More than half of overweight and obese people who lose weight through a diet and exercise regimen will regain it all within five years.[3]

Certainly, people can and do lose weight by changing their dietary patterns. Again, we distinguish between diet as a lifelong nutritional change and "diet" as a short-term, unsustainable, restrictive eating plan. You can lose weight with both, but only with the former can you keep it off long term and achieve real health gains. And, even with a lifelong diet, you must be aware of the biological changes that come with weight loss so you can counteract them when possible.

Your Metabolism and Diets

Our metabolism is the engine by which we burn caloric energy to power all bodily functions. To lose weight and gain health, we want that engine to be highly efficient. But, when the pounds start to come off, the metabolism machine slows down in an effort to conserve energy. This is good if we are starving, but not so good if we're attempting to lose extra weight.

Let's take a look at how our metabolism uses this energy. The *resting metabolic rate* (RMR) is the amount of energy we expend as human beings when we are at rest. It represents the energy required to maintain vital bodily functions such as breathing, heart rate, and blood pressure. Your brain uses about 19 percent of this resting energy, your liver about 27 percent, and your heart about 10 percent. Resting metabolic rate accounts for approximately 60-75 percent of our *total energy expenditure* (TEE) each day.[4]

So, what about the other 25–40 percent of our TEE? That is used in a couple of ways. The energy required to digest and absorb food (called the thermic effect of feeding) provides another 5–10 percent, and energy we use moving around (the thermic effect of activity) comprises about 20–30 percent.

The metabolic rate is important because the higher the rate, the more calories you're burning. The goal is to see if you can maintain or increase your metabolism in order to burn more calories. The problem is that when you start restricting calories, your resting metabolic rate lowers in response, and the more drastic the calorie restriction, the more drastic the drop.

That explains why people will initially lose weight with calorie restriction. But, when the body accommodates and lowers the metabolic rate, you burn fewer calories—causing a leveling off of weight loss, or *weight plateau*. And, as if that were not enough, when individuals start to restrict calories, the body also compensates by releasing a series of hormones that increase appetite and the drive to seek food. For every action we take to try and lose weight, there is a reaction by the body to adapt and regain it.

What's My RMR?

There are factors that contribute to what any one person's metabolic rate is. And, the less fat and more lean body mass you have at any weight, the higher your metabolic rate. In general, the rule of thumb is to multiply your weight by 10 to get an approximate number of calories that is your resting metabolic rate. As your body fat percentage goes up, your metabolic rate actually drops even if your weight stays steady. A skin caliper test, which measures skin folds at various parts of the body, is the simplest and most cost effective way to measure body fat.

So, two people who weigh the same amount are not necessarily burning the same number of calories—it's based on their own genetic metabolism and levels of body fat. If you weigh 180 pounds and you have 20 percent body fat, you are burning 1,800 or even 1,900 calories. But, the same person who has 40 percent body fat may only be burning 1,600 calories.

In addition, research has shown us that different populations have different metabolisms. For example, we know both African-American men and women have lower resting metabolic rates than their white peers.[5, 6]

And, we also know that as you get older and body fat tends

to increase while you burn fewer calories, it's harder to sustain your weight. If you do maintain your weight as you get older, the paradox is that you're actually getting fatter because most of us are losing a certain amount of muscle. So, in order for us to sustain weight as we get older, we actually have to eat less or exercise more to expend more energy.

Can We Change Our Metabolism?

The ultimate question is whether or not you really can change your metabolism significantly, and that's open to debate. The belief is that regular exercise and building of muscle can somehow alter your metabolism on a long-term basis, but even that is controversial.[7] So, it seems as though all of the forces in nature are working against us in trying to successfully lose weight. The only thing that we can actually do that makes any sense is to increase our physical activity.

It also makes sense to eat fewer calories, but not the kind of dramatic restriction that will be self-defeating by lowering your metabolic rate. It should only be a 500- to 700-calorie daily reduction. Shifting the nutrient makeup of those calories may be very useful as well, including lowering the carbohydrate percentage,[8] as is choosing more lower-glycemic carbs, which don't cause the spike in blood sugar and resulting release of insulin that high-glycemic carbs do. Examples of carbohydrate-containing foods with a low glycemic index (GI) include dried beans and legumes (such as kidney beans and lentils), all non-starchy vegetables, some starchy vegetables such as sweet potatoes, most fruit, and many whole grain breads and cereals (such as barley, whole wheat bread, rye bread, and all-bran cereal). Meats and fats don't have a GI because they do not contain carbohydrates. Chapter 11 has more information on eating for health and weight maintenance.

The Hormone Backlash

As mentioned previously, severe calorie restriction also triggers hormonal changes in our bodies. The gut (the stomach, intestines, and the rest of the digestive system) and the brain work in concert to satisfy the nutrient needs of the body. Food intake, appetite, and feelings of fullness are regulated by this gut/brain axis, and when the system believes it's being deprived of nutrients, it starts to make changes to compensate. It's a complex interaction involving our central nervous system and multiple sites within the brain itself that respond to a variety of different hormones being produced in the gut.[9] The end result is that when we cut calories dramatically and start to lose weight, ghrelin levels go up, triggering constant hunger, and leptin levels go down, decreasing the feeling of fullness.[10, 11]

There is good news in all of this. The discovery of these hormonal messengers and the pathways they travel has given us new targets for drug therapy. The science is advancing constantly (even as we write this book). Medicine is getting closer to the root causes of obesity and figuring out how to short circuit the hard wiring that "protects" us against sustained weight loss.

And, since we know that losing as little as 3–5 percent of total excess body weight can have an enormous impact on improving our health, severe calorie restriction is certainly unnecessary, as well as counterproductive. The goal is better health, and improving the quality of your diet with appropriate small reductions in calories will move you most effectively toward it. That goal may be better blood sugar control if you have diabetes, less pain if you have joint problems, improved sleep quality if you have apnea, or a reduction in medication if you have blood pressure and/or cholesterol problems.

Your Doctor's Role, Reframed

Your doctor (with the help of a good dietitian) can get you on the path to your diet for life. Eating for health should be supervised by healthcare professionals who can assess your metabolic rate and the calorie level you should reach to meet your daily energy goals.

This represents a fundamental shift for many doctors, who have left nutritional guidance for weight loss to the commercial self-help world. But, your weight and the health problems it causes you are a medical issue that needs medical oversight. You should have a full assessment and develop customized goals and action steps that work for you, including a dietary plan for life. We'll go through this in detail in chapter 10.

This shift toward physicians taking the lead in helping patients lose weight is an important one. Clinical research has proven that when an overweight adult is told by their doctor they should lose weight, they are significantly more likely to actually take action on that advice compared to peers whose doctor did not offer any weight advice.[12] That may sound kind of obvious, but too often weight is not addressed in the examining room. Sometimes this is because the doctor doesn't feel the patient will act on his advice, and sometimes it's because the patient doesn't seem open to the discussion. You can do your part by giving your doctor permission to talk to you about your weight and the impact it's having on your health.

Jill, Revisited

Jill is a motivated patient. She's not a fan of prescription drugs and would like to be able to go off the ACE inhibitor she is on to manage her hypertension. When Jill relates her eating patterns, which are heavy in restaurant and fast food fare, it's clear her sodium intake is probably also contributing to her hypertension. I refer her to a registered dietitian to come up with a meal plan that fits Jill's lifestyle, cuts down on the sodium, and promotes a healthy level of weight loss. She also pledges to join her daughter, who is an avid cyclist, in a daily exercise routine.

Six months later, Jill has dropped 12 pounds. Her blood pressure, while still above normal, has also improved, and I write her a new prescription at a much lower dose. We are both encouraged by the progress she's made and schedule a return visit in six months.

References

1. Jouanna J. *Greek Medicine from Hippocrates to Galen: Selected Papers*. BRILL, 2012.
2. Nicklas JM, Huskey KW, Davis RB, Wee CC. Successful weight loss among obese U.S. adults. *Am J Prev Med*. 2012 May; 42(5): 481–5.
3. Sarwer DB, von Sydow Green A, Vetter ML, Wadden TA. Behavior therapy for obesity: Where are we now? *Curr Opin Endocrinol Diabetes Obes*. 2009 Oct; 16(5): 347–52. doi: 10.1097/MED.0b013e32832f5a79.
4. Danforth E. Dietary induced thermogenesis: Control of energy expenditure. *Life Sci* 1981; 28: 1821–1827.
5. Weyer C, Snitker S, Bogardus C, Ravussin E. Energy metabolism in African Americans: Potential risk factors for obesity. *Am J Clin Nutr*. 1999 Jul; 70(1): 13–20.
6. Shook RP, Hand GA, et al. Low fitness partially explains resting metabolic rate differences between African American and white women. *Am J Med*. 2014 May; 127(5): 436–42.
7. Thompson JL, Manore MM, Thomas JR. Effects of diet and diet-plus-exercise programs on resting metabolic rate: A meta-analysis. *Int J Sport Nutr* 1996; 6: 41–61.

8. Ebbeling CB, Swain JF, Feldman HA, et al. Effects of dietary composition on energy expenditure during weight-loss maintenance. *JAMA*. 2012; 307(24): 2627–2634.

9. Acosta A, Abu Dayyeh BK, Port JD, Camilleri M. Recent advances in clinical practice challenges and opportunities in the management of obesity. *Gut*. 2014 Apr; 63(4): 687–95.

10. Maclean PS, Bergouignan A, Cornier MA, Jackman MR. Biology's response to dieting: The impetus for weight regain. *Am J Physiol Regul Integr Comp Physiol*. 2011 Sep; 301(3): R581–600.

11. Sumithran P, Prendergas LA, Delbridge E, et al. Long-term persistence of hormonal adaptations to weight loss. *N Engl J Med*. 2011; 365(17): 1597–1604.

12. Bish CL, Blanck HM, Serdula MK, Marcus M, Kohl HW, Khan LK. Diet and physical activity behaviors among Americans trying to lose weight: 2000 behavioral risk factor surveillance system. *Obes Res*. 2005; 13: 596–607.

Tips for Talking to Your Doctor

What's my resting metabolic rate?

_____

_____

_____

_____

_____

_____

How much weight do you think I need to lose to improve my health (e.g., blood pressure, diabetes, cholesterol levels, apnea, joint pain, etc.)?

_____

_____

_____

_____

_____

_____

CHAPTER 6

Fit but Fat:
A New Paradigm

Ken's Story

Ken is a 26-year-old, 6'3" male who makes his living as a professional athlete. During the playing season, Ken weighs 315 pounds. According to the charts, this gives him a morbidly obese body mass index of 39; however, as an athlete he is highly conditioned and has a significant amount of muscle mass, so in his case the BMI is not a very useful measurement of his health.

During the preseason and playing season, Ken is in fighting shape. He trains daily and sticks to a strict meal plan dictated by team staff. But, once the season ends, his trouble begins. Ken is unmarried and spends most of his time off traveling, doing speaking engagements, charity dinners, and corporate events. There's a lot of time spent in airplanes and airports, and plenty of rich food and free-flowing alcohol. As a result, Ken inevitably gains 20–30 pounds in the off-season, and each time it's harder to shake off when training starts again.

This year, Ken's season ended early due to a shoulder injury, and the weight gain was accompanied by a slight rise in blood pressure that has scared him into my office. Ken's body is his livelihood, and he wants to get the weight off and, most importantly, the blood pressure down, before the season starts up again.

Health at Every Size

While numbers such as BMI and weight are important, they certainly don't tell the whole story about your health, at least in isolation. People who are considered overweight by these measures may be very fit and not be experiencing any ill health effects. We know that healthy heart and lung function—*cardiorespiratory fitness*— achieved by regular exercise is a key marker of health. We also know that muscular fitness appears to be protective against elevated bad cholesterol (LDL) levels, which is a risk factor for heart disease and type 2 diabetes.[1]

As a doctor, my goal for your care has to be more than weight loss for aesthetics; it has to be weight loss for a health reason. The focus is fitness, not pounds. We are really focusing on improvements in overall health, whether it's mental health or physical health.

Patients come in and they may be 30 pounds overweight, but their blood pressure, cholesterol, and blood sugar are all normal. Does this mean that their weight is not a problem? If they are active and report that they exercise regularly, it may not be (although we might caution them against gaining additional weight).

But, if the patient leads a mostly inactive (sedentary) lifestyle, there is reason to be concerned about their future health. Just because they have yet to experience any ill health effects from their weight does not mean they won't in six months or a year. Most people don't go from being perfectly healthy to being ill. There is a transition period, a period of pre-disease (premorbidity), between wellness and illness. It's likely that most people who are overweight and inactive will develop hypertension, high blood sugar, and other obesity-related illnesses at some point unless they increase their fitness level and/or reduce their weight. We want to make certain we don't give people a false sense of optimism just because they happen to not have diabetes even though they are 30 pounds overweight.

So, as you see, exercise plays a large role in our state of health. Even if we have excess fat on our bodies, regular activity counteracts some of the ill effects and risk factors that fat brings with it. Studies have shown us that overweight people who are active and have high levels of cardiorespiratory fitness have lower death and disease (morbidity) rates than their inactive counterparts.[2, 3]

Fit but Fat

A "fit but fat" person is considered overweight or obese on the BMI charts but is metabolically healthy and without weight-related health issues. This is typically someone who exercises regularly, who doesn't carry mostly visceral fat, and who has a high level of cardiorespiratory fitness.

What is cardiorespiratory fitness? Essentially, it's how your heart and lungs work together to establish overall fitness. Cardiorespiratory fitness is achieved by moving large muscle groups for extended periods of time—in short, by regular exercise.

This type of fitness is a primary predictor of cardiovascular events and death.[4] We know that people of any size who have a low level of cardiovascular fitness are at a higher risk of dying—not only from cardiovascular disease, but from all causes—than those who are fit. Even someone considered obese by BMI may be protected against heart attack and stroke if they have a high level of cardiorespiratory fitness.[5]

Numbers Beyond the Scale

So, how do we assess someone who is overweight to determine if they have, or are at risk for, health problems? Today we can be much more sophisticated in what we're measuring beyond weight. We look at other measures of body composition, as well as blood tests that help us assess your level of fitness. Following are a few of the basic tests used to evaluate your health and fitness in the doctor's office.

Table 1. Body Mass Index and Weight Status	
BMI	**Status**
<19	Underweight
19 to 24.9	Normal
25 to 29.9	Overweight
30 to 39.9	Obese
≥40	Morbid obesity

- *Body mass index (BMI)*. The BMI is a measure of body fatness calculated from a person's height and weight. It is used to screen adults and children for potential weight problems and is used in population studies. The BMI does have limitations, however. Because it doesn't discern between fat and lean tissue, it is frequently inaccurate in athletes. It is also inconsistent across different ages and races. Still, it's a useful starting point for many people for determining if their weight is at a point where it could lead to health issues. Table 1 lists the BMI cut-off points for overweight and obesity. (See page 39 for a BMI chart.)

- **Waist circumference.** As discussed in chapter 3, fat that gathers in the abdominal region (visceral fat) carries additional health risk due to the inflammatory chemicals it pumps out. Women with a waist circumference of 35 inches or more and men with a waist circumference of 40 inches or more have a higher risk of health problems.
- **Body fat percentage.** As you might guess, this is the percentage of fat mass in your body versus your total body mass. Where the BMI is not very effective for athletes or highly conditioned people, the body fat percentage is a more useful measurement of fatness. A skin caliper test, which measures skin folds at various parts of the body, is the simplest and most cost effective way to measure body fat. But, there are other methods of calculating this value, including X-ray, underwater weighing, and others. Women should have a body fat percentage of 31 percent or less and men should be at 25 percent or less.
- **Blood tests.** If a person is overweight or obese, screening for health conditions related to excess weight makes sense. Blood tests include cholesterol, hemoglobin A1C (a measure of blood sugar), C-reactive protein (an inflammatory marker), and liver function.
- **Blood pressure.** Because excess weight is a significant risk factor for hypertension, it's important to keep an eye on blood pressure in overweight people.

I always emphasize with patients that progress is made when progress is measured. It's important that we get all these measurements down so that we can track them as the patient moves toward their goal of better health. In addition, it's important that they follow their progress at home. There are all kinds of fitness tracking devices available and multiple apps that help evaluate your fitness level (see "Additional Resources" for a list).

Tests are just one part of the equation. In order to establish your level of fitness and health goals, your doctor should perform a full assessment, including discussing your health and weight history, your lifestyle needs, and any barriers to care. We'll talk more about what that is and how to work with your doctor in chapter 10.

Healthy Eating and Movement

If you fall into the category of "fit but fat," you should be proud of your achievements. Exercise is a tremendous challenge; less than half of American adults meet the recommended physical activity guidelines for aerobic activity, and a dismal 20 percent meet both aerobic and muscle-strengthening activity goals.[6]

People overestimate how much they exercise by about 50 percent, just as they underestimate how much they eat by about 50 percent. So, any "fitness prescription" needs to have some discipline around it. Writing down or electronically tracking exercise, in addition to making a commitment to exercise most days of the week, is important for everyone. The U.S. Department of Health and Human Services says that adults need 150 minutes of moderate-intensity aerobic activity or 75 minutes of vigorous-intensity aerobics each week, along with muscle-strengthening activities two or more days a week.[7]

While losing excess weight isn't crucial if you are healthy and fit, maintaining the weight you are at is an important goal. Adding extra pounds will increase your risk and may make staying fit harder. So diet (as a lifestyle, not a quick fix) is important, along with continued exercise. I emphasize a sustainable long-term eating program, one that my patients can live with and stick to for life, because I do believe that the nutrient value of the foods you eat and your body's ability to absorb those nutrients are two of the most important determinants of how healthy you're going to be.

And we are recognizing that there is no single eating program that is significantly more successful than others. Once again, one size doesn't fit all. I prefer and recommend a lower carbohydrate, lower glycemic index diet because there is good evidence it works and I've seen it work, but there are plenty of other acceptable variations with solid clinical evidence behind them, such as the Mediterranean diet and the DASH diet. [8, 9, 10]

The main criteria are that the eating program selected is nutrient dense and satisfies your lifestyle needs. Whether you are overweight or not, you still have to eat well. I make the same recommendations to people who are not overweight. The only difference is a mild decrease of just a few hundred calories in those who are overweight. This is important, because as we discussed in chapter 5, the body responds to severe caloric restriction by initiating biologic events that then sabotage you.

Fighting the Stereotypes

There is such a stigma associated with obesity in our society. Someone carrying extra weight is automatically deemed unhealthy, as well as lacking willpower and motivation. The notion that someone can be physically fit and overweight is not yet widely accepted, just as many still have difficulty grasping the idea that a weight problem is biological instead of a character defect. We need to change those attitudes.

The medical profession also has to be careful in how they address patients who are overweight. Scolding or scare tactics are rarely effective. If a patient is overweight, but reports exercising regularly and has no signs of cardiovascular or metabolic health issues, they should be commended on their level of fitness and encouraged to keep up their efforts. Weight loss should not be a focus unless weight is causing the patient mental distress.

At the same time, it is important to keep a close eye on those overweight patients who are healthy "by the numbers," but who report being inactive, and to explain the link between inactivity, excess weight, and significant health problems in the future. And, for those who have other poor health habits who have the potential to increase weight and decrease overall health—such as inadequate sleep, use of alcohol and drugs, poor dietary patterns, and stress—developing strategies to deal with them is important. If this sounds like you, you should be seeing your doctor more often and setting goals to enhance your wellness and decrease your risk for obesity-related diseases.

Ken, Revisited

Skin caliper testing revealed that Ken's body fat percentage was at 15 percent, which put him solidly in the "fit" range. But, the rise in blood pressure was concerning to us both, as was the fact that Ken's LDL (bad) cholesterol was mildly elevated. Discussion of his family history revealed a history of hypertension and atherosclerosis (buildup of plaque in the arteries) in his family. And it was clear that his off-season food choices weren't helping.

We talked about Ken's off-season barriers to eating better and working out. When Ken was outside of the structured environment of training and team advisors, he would eat whatever was given to him. This proved to be a problem given the number of banquets and food-filled events he attended. He didn't have the time or knowledge to arrange for healthier food to be provided. So, he took the step of hiring a smart and resourceful registered dietitian as a full-time assistant to do the legwork for him. If a facility couldn't provide healthy foods he could eat (and it turned out that most could accommodate him), they would arrange to have a meal made and sent in. And he worked with his trainer to develop a series of "on the road" workouts he could squeeze in when traveling.

Hiring a full-time employee isn't a solution most people can afford, but it made sense for Ken. Even if you aren't a professional athlete, you can use the strategy of consulting a registered dietitian to educate yourself on smart food choices, and insurance often pays for the sessions.

By the time Ken headed back to preseason training, he was 10 pounds lighter and his blood pressure had dropped back down into the normal range. The team doctor and trainers were impressed by the strides he had made; he was in better preseason shape than he had been since starting for the team. And, he's scheduled his dietitian to come back on the payroll as soon as the season ends.

References

1. Kosola J, Ahotupa M, Kyröläinen H, Santtila M, Vasankari T. Good aerobic or muscular fitness protects overweight men from elevated oxidized LDL. *Med Sci Sports Exerc*. 2012 Apr; 44(4): 563–8.
2. Barlow CE, Kohl HW, Gibbons LW, Blair SN. Physical fitness, mortality and obesity. *Int J Obes Relat Metab Disord*. 1995; 19(Suppl 4): S41–4.
3. Loprinzi P, Smit E, Lee H, Crespo C, Andersen R, Blair SN. The "fit but fat" paradigm addressed using accelerometer-determined physical activity data. *N Am J Med Sci*. 2014 Jul; 6(7): 295–301.
4. Mcauley PA, Artero EG, Sui X, Lavie CJ, Almeida MJ, Blair SN. Fitness, fatness, and survival in adults with prediabetes. *Diabetes Care*. 2014 Feb; 37(2): 529–36.
5. Lee CD, Blair SN, Jackson AS. Cardiorespiratory fitness, body composition, and all-cause and cardiovascular disease mortality in men. *Am J Clin Nutr*. 1999 Mar; 69(3): 373–80.
6. U.S. Department of Health and Human Services. National Center for Health Statistics. *Health, United States, 2013: With Special Feature on Prescription Drugs*. Hyattsville, MD. 2014.
7. U.S. Department of Health and Human Services. *2008 Physical Activity Guidelines for Americans*. Washington, DC, 2008.
8. Soeliman FA, Azadbakht L. Weight loss maintenance: A review on dietary related strategies. *J Res Med Sci*. 2014 Mar; 19(3): 268–75. Review.
9. Dubnov-Raz G, Berry EM. Dietary approaches to obesity. *Mt Sinai J Med*. 2010 Sep–Oct; 77(5): 488–98. doi: 10.1002/msj.20210. Review.
10. Liebman M. When and why carbohydrate restriction can be a viable option. *Nutrition*. 2014 Jul–Aug; 30(7-8): 748–54.

Tips for Talking to Your Doctor

What are my BMI, body fat percentage, and waist circumference? What do these numbers mean?

_____

_____

_____

_____

_____

_____

I exercise at least three hours a week, but my BMI says I'm overweight. Am I fit? Do I need to lose weight for health purposes?

_____

_____

_____

_____

_____

_____

CHAPTER 7

Drugs and Weight

A Word from Dr. Lamm

Drug treatment is an essential option in the management of obesity. All doctors need to start thinking of the management of obesity in the same way we would high cholesterol or hypertension and consider weight loss drugs part of our treatment arsenal. We have a more limited group of medications for obesity than we do for these other conditions, but that will be changing over time as obesity science advances.

Physicians should familiarize themselves with both the science of these medications and the art of how to prescribe them. Combining medications may be the most effective approach, just like it is in other disorders. But, unlike other disorders, in obesity many of these medications seem to lose their potency over time as the body adjusts to their action. So, it's important to cycle medications, as well as use drug holidays. Finally, it's also critical to be very familiar with the drugs that promote weight gain. Removing those medications may be all that's necessary to make a clinically significant reduction in a patient's weight.

Norman Sussman, MD, psychiatrist and director of the treatment-resistant depression program at the NYU School of Medicine, is a colleague of mine at NYU Langone Medical Center. He is very familiar with the "art and science" of how the new obesity drugs work, as well as being a recognized expert in psychopharmacology—the study of the effects of drugs on mood and behavior. I've asked Dr. Sussman to share his considerable knowledge and experience on the role of medication in weight management.

Medication: A Double-Edged Sword

Medication plays a dual role in managing weight and weight-related health problems. On one hand, there are medicines that can help us lose weight by changing our appetite and the way our body processes food and energy. And on the other, there are medicines prescribed for chronic health conditions that actually cause us to gain weight as a side effect. As you work toward your goal of a healthy weight, understanding how medication can hurt and help your efforts is important.

Drugs that Promote Weight Gain

Let's start with the negative role drugs can play in weight management. There are many prescription and over-the-counter drugs that fuel weight gain. They do this in a variety of different ways. Some drugs may increase your appetite, promoting overeating. Others may decrease your energy levels or cause symptoms such as shortness of breath that make it difficult to exercise and burn calories. Then there are drugs that actually change the way your body uses and stores energy. They may slow your metabolism or alter how your body processes sugar (glucose) and stores fat.

It's an unfortunate reality that many drugs that are prescribed for weight-related health conditions—such as diabetes and heart disease—promote further weight gain and can lead to a vicious cycle of worsening symptoms and the need for more drugs. The same can be said for antidepressants; people who are obese have a higher incidence of depression. Some antidepressants may have weight gain side effects, which can worsen the depression. But we also know that when left untreated, depression and anxiety can lead to poor eating and sedentary behaviors that also fuel weight

Table 2. Drugs and Medications Associated with Weight Gain

Drug Class	Generic	Brand Name*
Antidepressants	amitriptyline, doxepin, fluvoxamine, imipramine, mirtazapine, nortriptyline, paroxetine, sertraline, escitalopram, citalopram, trimipramine	Adapin, Aventyl, Dilenor, Elavil, Endep, Luvox, Pamelor, Paxil, Remeron, Sinequan, Surmontil, Tofranil, Vanatrip, Zoloft, Lexapro, Celexa
Antihistamines	diphenhydramine, cyproheptadine	Aler-Dryl, Benadryl, Diphenhist, Siladryl, Silphen, Sominex, Unisom, other generic brands Periactin
Antipsychotics	chlorpromazine, clozapine, fluphenazine, haloperidol, loxapine, olanzapine, quetiapine, risperidone	Clozaril, FazaClo, Oxilapine, Risperdal, Seroquel, Thorazine, Zyprexa, other generic brands
Antiseizure/ anticonvulsants	carbamazepine, gabapentin, valproic acid	Carbatrol, Depakote, Epitol, Equetro, Horizant, Neurontin, Stavzor, Tegretol
Beta-blockers	atenolol, metoprolol, propranolol	Inderal, InnoPran, Lopressor, Pronol, Tenormin, Toprol
Contraception	estrogen, progestogens	Various
Corticosteroids	cortisone, prednisone, budesonide, ciclesonide, fluticasone	Alvesco, Flovent, Prednisone Intensol, Pulmicort, Sterapred
Diabetes — insulin	insulin aspart, insulin detemir, insulin glargine, insulin glulisine, insulin lispro, NPH (N), regular (R)	Apidra, Humulin, Humalog, Levemir, Lantus, Novolin, NovoLog
Diabetes — oral medications	chlorpropamide, glipizide, glimepiride, glyburide, pioglitazone, rosiglitazone, tolbutamide	Actos, Amaryl, Avandia, DiaBeta, Diabinese, Glucotrol, Glynase, Micronase, other generic brands
Mood stabilizers	lithium	Eskalith, Lithobid

*All brand names are registered trademarks of their respective owners.

gain. Fortunately, not all antidepressant drugs make people gain weight, and it's really a matter of working with your doctor to find a drug that is effective in alleviating depression while having a manageable number of side effects.

The medications listed in Table 2 are associated with weight gain. If you have been prescribed any of these, it's important to talk to your doctor about how they may be impacting your weight. In some cases, a dosage adjustment may be recommended, or your doctor may recommend a medicine in the same drug class that isn't associated with weight gain.

Among these drugs, some are more likely to cause weight gain and also are more likely to cause a greater amount of increase in body weight. The worst offenders are Zyprexa, Clozaril, Remeron, and Paxil. Nevertheless, if you never had a problem with weight before starting any drug, but find yourself gaining excess weight, it is safe to assume that it is a side effect of treatment.

Are Weight Loss Drugs Right for You?

Now that you know whether or not your prescriptions are promoting weight gain, let's talk about how drugs can actually help you lose weight. First, it's important to realize that there is no "magic pill" that can help you lose a significant amount of weight and keep it off without making other changes in your life as well—including moving more and eating healthy nutrient-dense foods.

Generally speaking, people who are successful with weight loss drugs are those who have a BMI of 30 or more (or a BMI of 27 or more with an associated weight-related health condition such as diabetes, hypertension, or heart disease) and who have been unable to lose or maintain weight loss with lifestyle change alone. These people have already made efforts in "diet and exercise" and have been unsuccessful, but they also understand that they must make permanent lifestyle changes in what they eat and how physically active they are for a weight loss pill to work long term.

If you fit this profile, a weight loss drug may be helpful to you. You also need to have realistic expectations about weight loss goals and outcomes. With today's current drugs, you should expect only modest weight loss (i.e., 3–9 percent of total body weight at one year).[1] But, as we know, even this modest weight loss can be enough to have a tremendous health benefit, which is the goal.

There are some people who may fit this profile, but who probably aren't good candidates for weight loss drugs for other reasons. If you are pregnant or breastfeeding, have unstable heart disease, have uncontrolled hypertension (higher than 180/110 mmHg), have a history of anorexia, have an unstable psychiatric disorder, or take a drug that is known to interact with weight loss drugs (e.g., MAO inhibitors, migraine drugs, adrenergic drugs), you should look at other treatment options. People who have certain types of glaucoma may also not be good candidates for weight loss drugs. Your healthcare provider should be aware of your full health history and current prescription and non-prescription drug use before putting you on a weight loss drug.

Today's Weight Loss Drugs

As of late 2014, there are only a handful of FDA-approved weight loss drugs available for the treatment of obesity. Let's take a look at each medication, its effectiveness, and the risks and benefits associated with each.

Diethylpropion (Tenuate)

Tenuate is one of the oldest weight-regulating drugs on the market. An appetite suppressant, it was approved as treatment for obesity in 1959. It works by stimulating the release of the central nervous system hormone norepinephrine and is intended for short-term use of 12 weeks or less because of its abuse potential.

One 2009 study looking at longer-term use of the drug found that after six months, subjects taking diethylpropion achieved an average of a 9.8 percent loss of initial body weight, and clinically significant weight loss continued at one year.[2]

It is also considered to have a high safety profile, in part due to how quickly the drug is excreted into the urine. Potential common side effects of Tenuate include nervousness, tremor, insomnia, headache, dry mouth, sweating, nausea, constipation, and thirst. Rarely, atrial fibrillation, pulmonary hypertension, and hallucinations may occur.

Phentermine

Like Tenuate, phentermine was first approved as an appetite suppressant in 1959 and is currently sold under the brand names Adipex-P, Ionamin, and a few others. Also similar to Tenuate, it works by stimulating norepinephrine release.

Side effects of phentermine include tachycardia, dry mouth, insomnia, and heart palpitations. The drug is designed for short-term use (12 weeks or less) and is considered a controlled substance due to its addictive properties.

In the 1990s, phentermine gained popularity when it was marketed along with the drugs fenfluramine and dexfenfluramine as a weight loss combination known as "fen-phen." Both fenfluramine and dexfenfluramine were taken off the market in 1997 after they were associated with heart valve disease.[3]

But, researchers remain interested in studying phentermine's effectiveness in combination with other weight loss drugs, and it remains relevant today. In 2012, the FDA approved the first phentermine combination drug since fen-phen: Qsymia.

Phentermine/Topiramate ER (Qsymia)

Qsymia is a combination of two drugs associated with weight loss through separate mechanisms. Phentermine suppresses appetite, and topiramate (an anticonvulsant drug used in epilepsy treatment) promotes feelings of fullness. Topiramate is also well known for changing the taste of foods and drinks, particularly with carbonated beverages. This side effect may also play a role in how Qsymia works to enable weight loss.

The drug is approved for adults with an initial BMI greater than 30 (obese), or BMI greater than 27 (overweight) with at least one weight-related health issue (e.g., high blood pressure, type 2 diabetes, abnormal amount of cholesterol and/or fat in the blood). Like most other weight loss drugs, it should be used in conjunction with a reduced-calorie diet and exercise. In clinical trials of the drug, subjects taking Qsymia maintained a mean weight loss of 17–22 pounds one year after starting it.[4, 5]

Qsymia is a controlled substance with the potential for abuse and addiction. Reported side effects of the drug include mood disorders, tingling, dizziness, distortion of taste, sleeplessness, constipation, dry mouth, kidney stones, metabolic acidosis, and glaucoma.[6]

Qsymia should not be taken by pregnant women, as use of the drug is associated with a fivefold increased risk of having a baby with a cleft palate. Because of this fact, it is only available through certified pharmacies that are enrolled in the Qsymia-certified pharmacy network.

Lorcaserin (Belviq)

Lorcaserin, known by the brand name Belviq, was approved by the U.S. Food and Drug Administration (FDA) in 2012 and introduced to the U.S. market the following year. It's thought that the drug works by stimulating the part of the brain that regulates appetite and it may promote weight loss through feelings of fullness. In clinical trials, subjects who took Belviq for two years sustained an average weight loss of 12 pounds.[7]

Belviq has very few side effects. The most commonly reported is headache. Other less common side effects include dizziness, fatigue, nausea, dry mouth, and constipation. People who have congestive heart failure or heart valve problems should be monitored very closely while taking Belviq.

Belviq is considered a controlled substance because users could develop psychiatric dependencies on the drug. Rarely, depression, anxiety, and suicidal thoughts were reported as side effects. It's very important to note that Belviq may cause dangerous interactions with a number of psychiatric drugs, including some antidepressants, mood stabilizers, and antipsychotic drugs.[8]

Naltrexone HCl and bupropion HCl (Contrave)

Contrave was approved by the FDA in September of 2014. A combination therapy believed to address both behavioral and physiological drivers of obesity, Contrave is approved for use in adults with a BMI of 30 or greater, or those with a BMI of 27 or greater who have at least one weight-related condition (e.g., type 2 diabetes, high cholesterol).

The medication combines an antidepressant (bupropion) with the anti-addiction drug naltrexone. Both of these drugs have a long history of use. Bupropion was approved under the brand name Wellbutrin in 1985 to treat depression and again in 1997 as Zyban, a smoking cessation aid. Naltrexone has been used to treat alcohol and opioid dependence since initial FDA approval in 1984. While Contrave's exact mechanisms of action aren't completely understood, it's thought that the drug works by regulating the dopamine reward system in the brain that controls cravings and overeating behaviors.

In Phase III trials of the drug, participants achieved weight loss of 6.1 percent of their body weight at one year. Reported side effects included nausea, constipation, headache, vomiting, dizziness, insomnia, dry mouth, and diarrhea.[9, 10]

Contrave is not recommended for use in patients with uncontrolled hypertension, as it can raise both blood pressure and heart rate. However, a large-scale study of Contrave users found that the drug did not raise the risk of heart attack.[11] Anyone prescribed Contrave should have both pulse and blood pressure regularly monitored. The FDA is requiring that the drug's manufacturer continue to assess long-term cardiovascular outcomes associated with Contrave use.

Orlistat (Xenical and Alli)

Orlistat blocks the absorption of up to one-third of the fat we eat. The prescription version of the drug, Xenical, was approved by the FDA in 1999. The drug is also available in a lower-dose, over-the-counter version—Alli—that was approved in 2007.

In addition to helping reduce weight an average of 11–18 pounds, orlistat has an added benefit of reducing LDL (bad) cholesterol levels.[12, 13] It has also been successful in lowering A1C in patients with diabetes.[14]

Among obese patients who meet the criteria for anti-obesity drug therapy, orlistat is most likely to benefit those who:

- do not feel hungry
- are not preoccupied with food
- eat out or order in often

- have increased cardiovascular disease risk or multiple cardiovascular risk factors
- are older
- take multiple medications.

The most troublesome side effects of orlistat are gastrointestinal. Because it blocks absorption of fat, it can result in diarrhea and fatty stools. This can be minimized by following a strict low-fat diet (<30 percent of diet). Another concern is the loss of fat-soluble vitamins with a potential for malnutrition. For this reason, a daily multivitamin containing vitamins A, D, E, and K is recommended.

Liraglutide (Saxenda)

Saxenda, a higher-dose (3 mg) version of liraglutide, was approved by the FDA in late 2014 as a treatment for obesity. Saxenda® (liraglutide [rDNA origin] injection) is indicated as an adjunct to a reduced-calorie diet and increased physical activity for chronic weight management in adult patients with an initial BMI of 30 or greater (obese) or 27 or greater (overweight) in the presence of at least one weight-related comorbid condition (e.g., hypertension, type 2 diabetes mellitus, or dyslipidemia).

In trials, average weight loss for those on the drug compared with placebo was 8 percent versus 2.6 percent. Among study participants, 64 percent of those taking liraglutide lost at least 5 percent of their body weight, and 33 percent lost at least 10 percent of their body weight.[15]

Patients on the drug also had huge improvements in obesity-related health measures, including blood pressure, cardiovascular risk biomarkers, lipids, and self-reported quality of life compared with those on placebo.

The drug has significant potential for improving the metabolic health of obese patients. In one study, a total of 61 percent of patients had prediabetes. The researchers found that a significantly higher proportion of this subgroup no longer showed any markers of prediabetes if they took liraglutide, compared with those on placebo (69 percent versus 33 percent). Among patients who didn't have prediabetes at the start of the study, significantly more of those taking placebo went on to develop the condition compared with those who were on liraglutide (21 percent versus 7 percent).[16]

Diabetes Drugs and Weight Loss Benefits

There are several drugs used in diabetes treatment that have the added benefit of promoting weight loss. While not currently approved for use as weight loss drugs, these medicines may also impact weight.

Metformin
Metformin was FDA approved for use in type 2 diabetes treatment in 1994. The drug is known to increase insulin sensitivity and facilitate weight loss; people who took metformin in the Diabetes Prevention Program (DPP) maintained an average 5.5 pound loss 10 years after the study concluded.[17] Because this amount of weight loss is relatively small and the drug can have significant gastrointestinal side effects (e.g., diarrhea, gas, stomach cramps), it has not been pursued as a primary treatment option for obesity. But, physicians may prescribe it in people who have prediabetes or other signs of metabolic disorders. It may also be prescribed in conjunction with drugs such as antipsychotics to counterbalance weight gain.

Insulin
As previously mentioned, injected insulin is often a cause of weight gain. However, a recent study showed that in some cases, inhaled (intranasal) insulin can reduce excess food in-

take by affecting feelings of fullness. Compared with a placebo, this type of insulin administration given after meals was shown to decrease appetite as well as reducing the intake of highly pleasant-tasting food, such as chocolate chip cookies. The inhaled insulin did not have this effect in the fasting, or before-meal, state.[18]

The study results suggest that inhaled insulin triggers brain changes that act as a fullness signal during the after-meal period, reducing the intake of tasty foods. Therefore, inhaled insulin taken after meals may be useful in preventing after-meal bingeing or snacking. It's important to note that the appetite suppression is not an approved use of Afrezza, the one inhaled insulin currently FDA approved in the United States. But, these study findings may have interesting implications for future development of inhaled insulin as an appetite suppressant.

Liraglutide (Victoza)

Liraglutide was approved as a blood sugar control agent for people with type 2 diabetes in 2010, before its more recent approval as a weight loss drug (see p. 98). The drug is a glucagon-like peptide-1 (GLP1) analogue and works on the body in several ways. First of all, it helps the beta cells of the pancreas produce insulin in response to blood glucose levels. It also helps slow digestion and acts as an appetite suppressant. All three of these mechanisms together result in weight loss and decreased insulin resistance. Clinically, liraglutide regulates appetite and food intake by decreasing hunger and increasing feelings of fullness after eating.

The Future of Weight-Management Drugs

The recent introductions of Belviq, Contrave, Saxenda, and

Qsymia to the weight loss drug market may mark a change for weight management in the United States. Before these FDA approvals started in 2012, we hadn't seen a new weight loss drug enter the market for well over a decade. This stagnation was, in part, due to the safety scare with fen-phen in the 1990s. In addition, Medicare and some private insurers have historically not covered these drugs, so cost can be an issue. As a result, the demand for and use of weight loss drugs have been lukewarm.

As the obesity epidemic reaches critical proportions, the healthcare community is recognizing that medications can play an important role for a growing portion of the population—those who would achieve significant health benefits from modest weight loss of around 5 percent. And, with building evidence of the safety and effectiveness of these drugs, there is a growing movement to get Medicare and private insurers to cover their cost.[19] As physicians, we need more "tools in our toolbox" to help these patients who need an added boost beyond nutritious eating and increased activity in order to lose weight and improve health. And, as obesity science advances, the hope is that we'll have even more of them from which to choose.

While medicine is a powerful tool that can improve the health of many people, it's important to remember that unless you commit to a foundation of proper eating and activity, these drugs won't help you achieve long-term benefits. As previously stated, these aren't "magic pills," but they may provide the extra push you need to make these healthy changes for life.

References

1. Yanovski SZ, Yanovski JA. Long-term drug treatment for obesity: A systematic and clinical review. *JAMA*. 2014 Jan 1; 311(1): 74–86. doi: 10.1001/jama.2013.281361. Review.
2. Cercato C, Roizenblatt VA, Leança CC, et al. A randomized double-blind placebo-controlled study of the long-term efficacy and safety of diethylpropion in the treatment of obese subjects. *Int J Obes* (Lond). 2009 Aug; 33(8): 857–65. doi: 10.1038/ijo.2009.124. Epub 2009 Jun 30.
3. FDA Announces Withdrawal Fenfluramine and Dexfenfluramine (Fen-Phen). September 15, 1997. http://www.fda.gov/Drugs/DrugSafety/PostmarketDrugSafetyInformationforPatientsandProviders/ucm179871.htm
4. Gadde KM, Allison DB, Ryan DH, et al. Effects of low-dose, controlled-release, phentermine plus topiramate combination on weight and associated comorbidities in overweight and obese adults (CONQUER): A randomised, placebo-controlled, phase 3 trial. *Lancet*. 2011; 377(9774): 1341–1352.
5. Allison DB, Gadde KM, Garvey WT, et al. Controlled-release phentermine/topiramate in severely obese adults: A randomized controlled trial (EQUIP). *Obesity* (Silver Spring). 2012; 20(2): 330–342.
6. Qsymia® (phentermine and topiramate extended-release) capsules CIV [Prescribing Information]. Mountain View, CA: VIVUS, Inc.; 2013.
7. Smith SR, Weissman NJ, AndersonCM, et al. Behavioral modification and lorcaserin for overweight and obesity management (BLOOM) Study Group. Multicenter, placebo-controlled trial of lorcaserin for weight management. *N Engl J Med*. 2010; 363(3): 245–256.
8. Mahgerefteh B, Vigue M, Freestone Z, Silver S, Nguyen Q. New drug therapies for the treatment of overweight and obese patients. *Am Health Drug Benefits*. 2013 Sep; 6(7): 423–30.
9. Wadden TA, Foreyt JP, Foster GD, et al. Weight loss with naltrexone SR/bupropion SR combination therapy as an adjunct to behavior modification: The COR-BMOD trial. *Obesity*. 2011; 19: 110–120.
10. Greenway FL, Fujioka K, Plodkowski RA, et al. COR-I Study Group. Effect of naltrexone plus bupropion on weight loss in overweight and obese adults (COR-I): A multicentre, randomised, double-blind, placebo-controlled, phase 3 trial. *Lancet*. 2010 Aug 21; 376(9741): 595–605.
11. Orexigen announces successful interim analysis of contrave light study. Orexigen Therapeutics Press Release. November 25, 2013. http://ir.orexigen.com/phoenix.zhtml?c=207034&p=irol-newsArticle&ID=1879629&highlight= Accessed 09/11/14.

12. Bray GA, Ryan DH. Update on obesity pharmacotherapy. *Ann N Y Acad Sci.* 2014 Apr; 1311: 1–13. doi: 10.1111/nyas.12328. Epub 2014 Mar 18. Review.
13. Florentin M, Tselepis AD, Elisaf MS, Rizos CV, Mikhailidis DP, Liberopoulos EN. Effect of non-statin lipid lowering and anti-obesity drugs on LDL subfractions in patients with mixed dyslipidaemia. *Curr Vasc Pharmacol.* 2010 Nov; 8(6): 820–30. Review.
14. Jacob S, Rabbia M, Meier MK, Hauptman J. Orlistat 120 mg improves glycaemic control in type 2 diabetic patients with or without concurrent weight loss. *Diabetes Obes Metab.* 2009 Apr; 11(4): 361–71. doi: 10.1111/j.1463-1326.2008.00970.x. Epub 2009 Jan 22.
15. Wadden TA, Hollander P, Klein S, et al. NN8022-1923 Investigators. Weight maintenance and additional weight loss with liraglutide after low-calorie-diet-induced weight loss: The SCALE maintenance randomized study. *Int J Obes* (Lond). 2013 Nov; 37(11): 1443–51.
16. Astrup A, Rössner S, Van Gaal L, et al. Effects of liraglutide in the treatment of obesity: A randomised, double-blind, placebo-controlled study. *Lancet.* 2009; 374(9701): 1606–1616.
17. Diabetes Prevention Program Research Group, Knowler WC, Fowler SE, Hamman RF, et al. 10-year follow-up of diabetes incidence and weight loss in the Diabetes Prevention Program Outcomes Study. *Lancet.* 2009 Nov 14; 374(9702): 1677–86. doi: 10.1016/S0140-6736(09)61457-4. Epub 2009 Oct 29.
18. Hallschmid M, Higgs S, Thienel M, Ott V, Lehnert H. Postprandial administration of intranasal insulin intensifies satiety and reduces intake of palatable snacks in women. *Diabetes.* 2012 Apr; 61(4): 782–9.
19. "Treat and Reduce Obesity Act" fact sheet. Obesity Action Coalition. http://www.obesityaction.org/treat-and-reduce-obesity-act. Accessed 9/13/14.

Tips for Talking to Your Doctor

Do any of the medicines I'm currently taking cause weight gain as a side effect? If so, are there other options for me? Can the dosage be changed or can another medicine be substituted?

_____

_____

_____

_____

_____

_____

Am I a candidate for any of the currently available weight loss drugs? Why or why not?

_____

_____

_____

_____

_____

_____

_____

_____

The Surgical Solution: Who Is a Candidate?

A Physician/Patient Story

I was always big. I come from a very athletic family; my parents were both super athletes and totally fit, and I was the first of seven children and for some reason I was just fat from the get-go. I went to my first doctor about losing weight when I was 10. Despite this, I had a good childhood—I was just stuck with my weight the whole time and so learned to use my size to my advantage, playing high-level rugby in Australia.

I became a surgeon before I turned 30 and had my own private practice by age 34. I became an expert at minimally invasive surgery and taught other surgeons around the world. And I began to perform bariatric surgeries, transforming people from obese and chronically ill to healthy and happy people leading normal lives. I found it to be some of the most satisfying work I've ever done, quite possibly because I recognized myself in many of the patients.

While I was leading a professionally satisfying life, the pain and humiliation of always being hungry and fighting it just exhausted me. I tried every diet and every weight loss pill. Over a 10-year period I lost 60–80 pounds five times. It would take me about a year to do it, through running and calorie control, but I always regained it. I just could not stop eating; I could never control hunger.

And that went on and on and on like an endless cycle and then one year, in 1999, I just got really sick and ended up with all the diseases that you get from obesity. At that point I was 42 and I was on 11 medicines. I was performing weight loss surgery myself by then and I realized I needed to help myself, so I went to a surgeon friend of mine in Australia and I had a Lap-Band®. I have lost about 120 pounds and kept it off for 15 years, and I have come off pretty much all of the medicine except for one blood pressure pill and one aspirin a day.

I am in good health and I weigh less now than I did when I was 15. I have been able to use my experience to help treat patients who are obese and educate them about the decision to have surgery and doing the right things postoperatively. I've made it work for many years now and they can see the end result of both the surgery and the commitment to eating right and staying active.

My experience also helps me understand the psychological side of obesity both before and after the surgery. It becomes a challenge for people to learn how to cope with actually not being fat and the reactions they will get from others. And the weight also has an effect on marriages and relationships and other aspects of life. I have operated on more than 8,000 people and it's been a joy to be able to help them.

What Is Bariatric Surgery?

Bariatric surgery is broken down into two main groups. First, there is the type where you make the size of the stomach smaller and that limits the amount of food a patient eats because they get full very quickly. Second, there is the malabsorptive type of operations where you eat, you have some degree of restriction, but you don't absorb it because your bowel is really shortened and you basically poop out what you eat.

By far the most common is the former, where we make the stomach smaller. There are three versions of this surgery: the bypass, the band, and the sleeve, which will be discussed in detail in the next chapter. But, no matter what the operation, it requires a fairly significant commitment from the patient.

How It Works

All these bariatric operations work by reducing the urge to eat and also by helping the patients get full more quickly and with less food. There is a thing called the satiety center in the hypothalamus of the brain that governs the urge to eat. Skinny people tend to eat only when they are hungry, they eat a moderate amount of food, and they get a sensation that they have had enough.

The problem with obese people is they never get that sensation, and people who are fat are basically hungry all day. They eat and they are never satisfied and never feel like they have had enough. So there is a huge transition that happens to these people when they have weight loss surgery. They feel that, number one, "I am not that hungry," and number two, "Wow, I just had that small meal and I feel like I have had enough." So it's those two feelings that make the difference rather than bariatric surgery being a restrictive and punitive blocking mechanism, which is a huge misconception about weight loss surgery.

There are about 50 recognized neurologic pathways that fire chemicals and hormones out to the brain, and they all come from about three or four segments at the top of the stomach. So, the three big operations that we do all affect that piece of the stomach, so these patients all get that wonderful feeling of being less interested in food and then being full and satisfied quicker.

Is It Right for You?

The goal of any bariatric surgery is to treat two things. First, we are treating disease that is caused or made worse by obesity in order to prevent further deterioration of a person's health. And second, we are doing it to increase their quality of life.

Who is a good candidate for bariatric surgery? Guidelines from the National Institutes of Health (NIH) state that if your BMI is greater than 40, or 35 to 39.9 with comorbid obesity-related conditions such as diabetes, sleep apnea, hypertension, hyperlipidemia, gastroesophageal reflux disease (GERD), asthma, and arthritis, you are a candidate for bariatric surgery.[1]

However, the NIH guidelines have not been updated in nearly 15 years, and based on newer studies we now know that people with lower BMIs may also be good candidates for bariatric surgery. The American Association of Clinical Endocrinologists, the Obesity Society, and the American Society for Metabolic and Bariatric Surgery issued comprehensive clinical practice guidelines for the bariatric surgery patient in 2013. These guidelines state that people with BMIs of 30–34.9 may also benefit from bariatric surgery if they have diabetes or metabolic syndrome and have been unable to lose weight other ways.[2]

There is a growing body of research that demonstrates the enormous benefits of bariatric surgery for morbidly obese people with type 2 diabetes. In these patients, the surgical alteration of the gastrointestinal (GI) tract actually changes the metabolic pathways and can put diabetes into remission, bringing blood sugar levels back to normal and also improving blood pressure and lipid levels.[3] These alterations in hormone secretion are so dramatic that, in some circles, the actual name of the procedure is now undergoing a change from bariatric to metabolic surgery.[4] We'll look at what types of surgery are most effective for diabetes in the next chapter.

In addition to meeting the BMI and health criteria, a patient must appreciate that this surgery is a tool that they can use, not a quick fix. They have to accept that without a long-term commitment to their other tools of eating healthy and moving more, the surgery will not work. They have to prepare for it in this way to make it work to its full extent. And, quite honestly, the vast majority of obese people are ready and willing to make this commitment. In my career, I have met very few people who haven't tried. One of the misconceptions out there about fat people is that they just don't try or care, and that's just nonsense.

The vast majority does try; they do care. But the standard mantra of "eat less and exercise more" just doesn't work for people of this size. So, if a patient walks in and they are morbidly obese with related health issues, and they have thought about it enough to come and make an appointment with us, then I'll talk to them about it. I'll outline what I think are the keys to make their surgery work, and if they are able to understand that, then I'll offer them an operation.

When Bariatric Surgery Isn't Your Best Option

There is no guaranteed success with bariatric surgery. As we've said, the people who succeed are the ones who understand the foundations and basics of healthy eating and of daily activity, or who are willing to learn them and implement change in their lives. However, that's never going to be 100 percent of people. Does that mean that if someone who is morbidly obese, who has diabetes, debilitating arthritis, and sleep apnea comes to us for surgical help, that we refuse them this potentially life-saving treatment because they cannot do those things? That's where the conundrum comes in.

The philosophy at our center is that we will try to help you make these changes with a comprehensive supportive program that educates you about how to eat and exercise and provides psychological support. But, you need to understand that you will not do well with surgery if you do not understand these issues and you do not come back and see a nutritionist and come to a support group. We always educate our patient and provide postoperative support, but we cannot force feed them.

Aside from these guidelines, there are a handful of other exclusionary criteria that may take surgery off the table for you, at least for a time. This includes if you are pregnant or lactating, if you have a serious uncontrolled psychiatric illness (including substance abuse and certain eating disorders), or if you have a health condition that isn't compatible with caloric restriction.

Getting in the Right Frame of Mind

The patients we see are usually quite desperate because they have tried many different diets and exercise and they tried to lose weight and either they haven't lost weight, or they lost weight and regained it. Often, before they will cover a bariatric procedure, health insurers will require that a patient "prove" their motivation and compliance by coming in once a month for six months and actively trying to lose weight. Even with people who have done that, it does not predict whether they will do well with surgery or not, because that's not really an accurate way of ascertaining the motivation compliance and the eventual ability to change their lifestyle.

We require a psychological assessment for potential patients. This is not so much to assess how well we think they will do postoperatively, for as we've said already, that is a very difficult thing to test. Instead, it's to help pick out people who may have serious undiagnosed psychological disorders such as depression or bipolar disease or schizophrenia, as these factors can influence obesity and would be important to treat appropriately before surgery could be considered.

Honestly, we get surprised every week. People about whom we may have been unsure may do really well, and people who we thought were going to do brilliantly don't, and so it's very hard to know ahead of time who is going to do well.

So, my attitude is that if you meet the criteria today and you are psychiatrically sound, this is an appropriate treatment.

Teamwork

It's not just surgeons who treat bariatric surgery patients. In our practice, we have two full-time registered dietitians, two full-time psychologists, and a social worker who runs our free patient support group. We encourage people to have therapeutic relationships. Not a psychologist, necessarily, but a counselor or a social worker or another trained professional. I think the disease of obesity is much more complicated than any other chronic medical disease that's out there and much more complicated than diabetes or hypertension, which are very difficult chronic diseases to manage.

Usually, a patient is sent to us from their internist or other primary care provider (PCP). You'll see in chapter 10 how Dr. Lamm evaluates and assesses each patient, then works with them to figure out the treatment option that's right for them.

When a patient ends up at our practice to discuss surgery, we try to work closely with the referring doctor to make sure we have all of the patient's health history and information and are sharing the relevant information back with the doctor.

We will also do our own comprehensive health history and interview with the patient to make sure we have all the information we need. If recent blood cholesterol and A1C tests have not been taken by the PCP, we will order these tests. Then, along with our team, we work with the patient to go through a series of screening procedures before surgery would actually take place. These include:

- *Clinical nutrition evaluation.* A registered dietitian (RD) evaluates current dietary habits and advises the patient on changes required following surgery.

- *Nutrient screening.* Blood tests can measure micronutrient levels to make sure there are no underlying issues and to assess whether supplementation is needed.
- *Gastrointestinal screening.* A patient who is considered at risk for or has a history of GI problems may undergo imaging studies and/or endoscopy.
- *A psychosocial-behavioral evaluation.* As discussed previously, this will screen for any psychiatric disorders. It also involves a patient-provider discussion to talk about any barriers to behavior change that face the patient at home and how to overcome them after the surgery.
- *Smoking cessation counseling.* Smokers need to quit at least six weeks before surgery, and kick the habit for good thereafter.
- *Pregnancy and contraception counseling.* Women who undergo bariatric surgery should avoid pregnancy for 12–18 months. In addition, some oral contraceptives may need to be discontinued before surgery to prevent blood clotting problems.

Other tests may be ordered depending on a patient's individual health history.

References

1. Practical guide to the identification, evaluation and treatment of overweight and obesity in adults. National Institutes of Health; National Heart, Lung and Blood Institute; North American Association for the Study of Obesity. October 2000.
2. Mechanick JI, Youdim A, Jones DB, et al., American Association of Clinical Endocrinologists, Obesity Society, American Society for Metabolic & Bariatric Surgery. Clinical practice guidelines for the perioperative nutritional, metabolic, and nonsurgical support of the bariatric surgery patient—2013 update: cosponsored by American Association of Clinical Endocrinologists, the Obesity Society, and American Society for Metabolic & Bariatric Surgery. *Endocr Pract.* 2013 Mar–Apr; 19(2): 337–72.
3. Tham JC, Howes N, le Roux CW. The role of bariatric surgery in the treatment of diabetes. *Ther Adv Chronic Dis.* 2014 May ;5(3): 149–57. doi: 10.1177/2040622313513313. Review.
4. Rubino F. From bariatric to metabolic surgery: Definition of a new discipline and implications for clinical practice. *Curr Atheroscler Rep.* 2013 Dec; 15(12): 369.

Tips for Talking to Your Doctor

Am I a candidate for bariatric surgery based on my BMI and other health conditions?

_____

_____

_____

_____

_____

_____

_____

If I choose bariatric surgery, what support and nutrition resources can you offer to help me through the process?

_____

_____

_____

_____

_____

_____

_____

CHAPTER 9

The Surgical Solution: How Bariatric Surgery Works

A Word from Dr. Lamm

I am fortunate enough to know and work with not just one, but two leading bariatric surgeons. Dr. Christine Ren-Fielding, MD, FACS, FASMBS, is Professor of Surgery at NYU School of Medicine and is considered by many to be the leading Lap-Band® surgeon in the United States, having performed more than 4,000 gastric band procedures. She is the founder and director of the NYU Langone Weight Management Program, and is the Chief of the Division of Bariatric Surgery. Dr. Ren-Fielding has been involved extensively in research in vascular medicine, angiogenesis, and bariatric surgery. In this chapter, she provides an expert look on how bariatric surgery works and what to expect after the procedure.

The Surgical Solution

For patients who are committed to changing, bariatric surgery offers a life-changing, and often life-saving, opportunity to dramatically improve their health. Study after study has shown us that bariatric surgery can significantly improve, and in some cases completely resolve, serious health conditions including type 2 diabetes, sleep apnea, high blood pressure, high cholesterol, GERD, joint problems, heart disease, and certain cancers.[1] It can reduce a person's risk of premature death from obesity-related conditions such as these by up to 40 percent.[2]

We say a patient must be committed because the surgery is not an "easy fix." Far from it, each patient must commit to permanent changes in the way they eat and move each day. And, as with any surgery, there are certain risks to consider.

The three most common bariatric procedures performed in America today are the gastric bypass, the sleeve gastrectomy, and the adjustable gastric band (or Lap-Band®). Gastric bypass is what is known as a malabsorptive procedure, in that it changes the way the digestive tract works and how nutrients are absorbed. Sleeve gastrectomy and adjustable gastric band are known as *restrictive procedures*, because they limit food intake by creating a smaller stomach for food to pass into.

Gastric Bypass

The most common bariatric weight loss operation in America is the gastric bypass, also called the Roux-en-Y procedure (after Swiss surgeon César Roux, who developed the procedure for the treatment of stomach ulcers over a century ago).

Surgically, we cut and separate the stomach at the very top to create a golf ball–sized piece of stomach (or pouch) to which we sew the intestine. So, the food comes into the golf ball stomach, goes down into the intestine, and bypasses the stomach and the duodenum completely (Figure 7).

Even though the surgery is known as gastric bypass, the mechanisms by which it triggers weight loss have a lot to do with the duodenum. The duodenum is the first section of the intestine that comes after the stomach. In a normal digestive tract, nutrients enter the duodenum and the nearby pancreas senses any sugars and carbohydrates and secretes insulin.

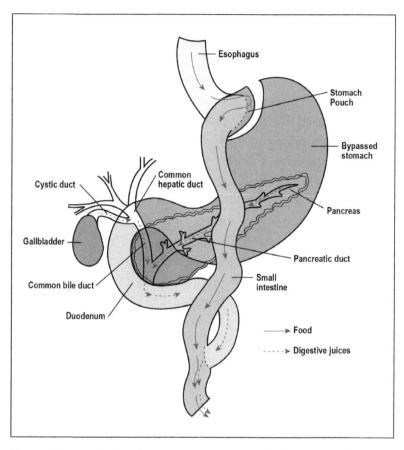

Figure 7. During the gastric bypass procedure, part of the stomach is detached from the rest, creating a small pouch. The pouch is connected to a lower part of the small intestine—an arrangement that resembles a Y. As a result, parts of the stomach and small intestine are bypassed. However, digestive juices (bile acids and pancreatic enzymes) can still mix with food, enabling the body to absorb vitamins and minerals, reducing the risk of nutritional deficiencies.

If nutrients are detoured away from the duodenum, the pancreas has a much more blunted reaction and it changes blood sugar very differently. This is why the gastric bypass procedure has a high success rate of symptom remission when performed on people with type 2 diabetes.

The duodenum is also where many gut hormones are stimulated and create a cycle of increased blood sugar. Once you take away food from the duodenum, the blood sugar stabilizes and a lot of those gut hormones don't get secreted.

The other thing that occurs is that caloric intake is drastically decreased due to the size of the stomach. So, people who are probably taking in 500 calories a day for the first three to six months have a drastic decrease in their appetite, they have minimal thirst, and they may actually feel a little nauseated.

When we eat, food enters our stomach where it gets mixed with water and acids, then is diluted and mechanically crushed, and then goes into the duodenum and intestines. Normal digestion is a slow process. After gastric bypass there is none of this settling in the stomach; undigested food goes directly into the intestines, and sometimes that doesn't feel so great. It certainly feels different and some people have a little bit of nausea afterward, which may last for a month or two until they acclimate, and then it typically goes away.

Surgical Complications

Gastric bypass is major abdominal surgery. All surgery carries a risk of infection, bleeding, and blood clots. There is also a risk of postoperative pneumonia. In addition to these general, short-term surgical complications, the following longer-term complications can develop weeks to months following the procedure:

- **Leak.** The suture or staple lines where the intestines are separated and connected could potentially not heal properly and leak into the abdominal cavity, which can lead to life-threatening sepsis. This typically occurs in the first several weeks after surgery.
- **Stricture.** The surgical connection between the

stomach pouch and intestine can form too much scar tissue and narrow significantly, which can block food and hydration. This would require an endoscopy to stretch the opening. This typically occurs 4–8 weeks after surgery.

- **Ulcers.** If a person smokes or takes large doses of nonsteroidal medications such as ibuprofen or aspirin, they are at increased risk for developing ulcers.
- **Hernia.** After a significant loss of fat in the abdomen, the intestine may twist and block itself. This is called an internal hernia and can cause intestinal blockage, which requires surgery to repair.
- **Gallstones.** Rapid weight loss can cause the development of gallstones, so we put patients on a short-term medication to decrease the risk of developing gallstones.

Nutritional Complications

The nutritional complications with gastric bypass are also pretty significant. The most common one is iron deficiency, particularly in menstruating, premenopausal women. Gastric bypass patients may also become deficient in calcium and protein.

In people without a bypass, the duodenum (the first section of the small intestine) is responsible for absorbing most of the iron, calcium, and protein from food. In gastric bypass patients, the duodenum is bypassed. The rest of the intestinal tract can absorb some of these nutrients, but it isn't very good at it. So, people with gastric bypass need to take iron and calcium supplements and make sure they eat enough protein in order to "overload" the rest of the intestine.

Vitamin B_{12} levels can also be low, because B_{12} is absorbed in the stomach in the presence of acid. When the size of the stomach is smaller and, consequently, so is the amount of acid in the stomach, B_{12} is affected.[3] So, we also recommend that gastric bypass patients take B_{12} supplements. Both Vitamin B_{12} and iron are important for making blood. If a patient is low in either of these nutrients, they can become anemic and have low blood levels, which may require iron infusions or a blood transfusion.

Outcomes

People who undergo gastric bypass lose an average of 62 to 68 percent of their excess body weight in the first year.[4] Weight loss typically levels off after two years, with an overall excess weight loss between 50 and 75 percent.[5] On average, patients will regain 20–25 percent of their weight within 10 years.[6] Gastric bypass, overall, is the most effective operation for people with long-term diabetes because of the positive effects it has on the pancreas and insulin secretion. It can lead to improvement or even remission of type 2 diabetes.

Sleeve Gastrectomy

The second most common bariatric surgery is called the sleeve gastrectomy. The name is a bit of a misnomer; there is no sleeve being put on the stomach. The procedure actually involves an amputation of 80 percent of the stomach (Figure 8)

The stomach is about the size of a small football and it has the shape of the left ear, so it's the earlobe portion of the stomach that actually stores the food while you are eating. The stomach fills up from the bottom up, so when the top of the stomach stretches it signals the brain; that's part of the fullness or satisfaction sensation. Sleeve gastrectomy involves cutting the earlobe portion of the stomach off lengthwise, so that a long skinny tube remains.

What is left looks like a sleeve, or a small banana or tube.

It works in two ways. First, it has a smaller capacity, so instead of eating three or four slices of pizza you are going to be full with one slice of pizza. Second, there is some evidence that the portion of the stomach removed, which is the storage part or the fundus, has cells that make the hunger hormone ghrelin. So, there is some evidence that if we remove this aspect of the stomach, we are decreasing the ghrelin that's being produced and therefore a patient is less hungry.

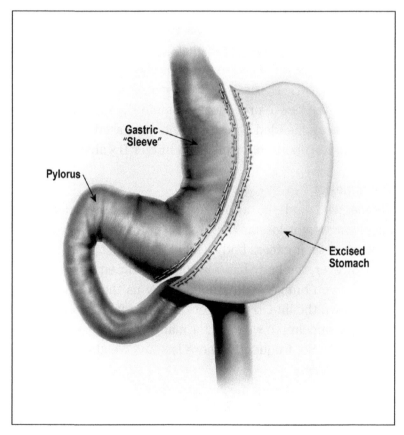

Figure 8. Vertical sleeve gastrectomy, known as the gastric sleeve. The procedure removes 80 percent of the stomach to limit its capacity for food.

Surgical Complications

Like gastric bypass, sleeve gastrectomy has the same risk of short-term surgical complications like bleeding, blood clots, infection, and pneumonia. There is also the risk of a staple line leak where the stomach is cut and sealed with titanium staples. Sometimes that staple line does not heal properly and if it pulls apart and creates a leak, it can cause an abscess that could be fatal if not treated. This typically occurs in the first several weeks.

Very rarely, if too much stomach is taken away and the remaining stomach tube is too narrow, then some people cannot eat or drink enough. They may lose too much weight and have trouble getting enough nutrients.

Unlike gastric bypass, there are very few nutritional problems with the sleeve procedure. Vitamin B_{12} supplementation may be recommended because of the decreased stomach acid following the operation, which can hinder B_{12} absorption.

Outcomes

People who undergo a sleeve gastrectomy generally have excellent weight loss at the onset. On average, they lose 65 percent of their excess body weight in the first year.[7]

However, the body has a lot of different emergency plans to make you hungry, and studies show us that three or four years down the line, the hunger-blunting effect of sleeve gastrectomy appears to wear off for many, and people do start to get hungry. So, frequently, there is some weight regain after the initial loss.

There are different mechanisms and pathways to stimulate people to hunger, and we are just beginning to understand them all. The good news is that if the patient has embraced a new relationship with healthy food and daily activity along the way, they will be more likely to keep the weight off in the long run.

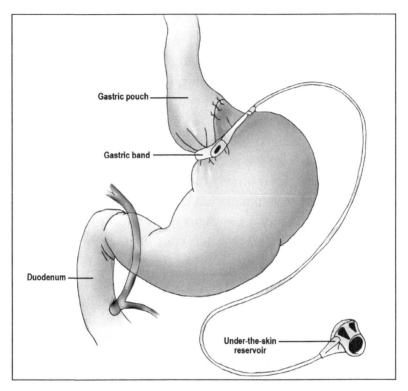

Figure 9. During adjustable gastric banding, an adjustable band is inserted through an incision and placed around the top of the stomach to create a small pouch. When the Lap-Band patient eats, food is restricted to this small pouch. This makes the patient feel full sooner, helping them to eat less.

Adjustable Gastric Banding (Lap-Band®)

Finally, we have the adjustable gastric band, which is also known by the trade name Lap-Band® (Figure 9). It is the least invasive operation that we have available, but it also requires the most teamwork toward making it work and keeping it working. What do I mean by that? Well, it's not just the surgeon doing the operation and not just the patient having the surgery, but the patient coming back for follow-up regularly afterward.

The band itself is made out of silicone, with a balloon on the inside. It's positioned around the very top of the stomach. The band is connected to a small reservoir with tubing, and that reservoir is placed under the skin in the abdominal wall.

When tightened, the band compresses the external walls of the stomach, and in doing so it also compresses a nerve called the vagus nerve that appears to interrupt some of the hunger signals from the stomach to the brain.

The band is not routinely tightened during the surgery itself. Each person is unique and requires a different amount of compression around the vagus nerve for the band to work effectively. It is similar to when your doctor starts you on a new medication, and you increase the dosages regularly and gradually until you get the full benefit from the drug. It's a process of fine-tuning the device to its full therapeutic benefit.

After the procedure, the patient comes in once a month for the first six to twelve months. Each time they come in, we talk about their symptoms and level of hunger, and based on their answers, we will either tighten their band, leave it alone, or loosen the band to get the right end result, which is a feeling of appetite suppression and self-regulated portion control (i.e., they feel full after eating small portions of food).

To tighten the band, we insert a special needle through the skin into the reservoir and inject saline solution that travels into the band to fill it and compress the stomach. The effect is very similar to a blood pressure cuff that tightens around your arm as the inflation bulb is squeezed.

Complications

Surgical complications from adjustable gastric banding are extremely rare, since the stomach and intestines are not cut and the band is placed using minimally invasive, or laparoscopic, surgical techniques. The most common complication is an incorrect fit of the band. The band may be too small for the person's stomach, and at the time of surgery it looks fine but afterward the patient has trouble drinking or eating. In this case, a bigger size band would need to be placed.

Longer-term (1–2 years after surgery) complications that can arise involve unintentional movement of the band. When we place it, it's just below the bottom of the esophagus, which is at the very top of the stomach. The band can shift downward on the stomach and if it does that, it's incorporating a greater diameter of the stomach, which makes the band very tight and can cause vomiting and reflux, particularly at night during sleep. Over time, excessive vomiting can lead to vitamin B_1 (thiamine) deficiency. This is called band slippage.

Another rare but potential long-term complication of adjustable gastric banding is called a *band erosion*. This occurs when the band actually rubs through the stomach wall and winds up on the inside lining of the stomach. The stomach heals itself behind where the band erodes in, so the area rarely becomes infected, but the band will stop working and requires a surgical procedure to remove the band, plus a second procedure to replace the band once the stomach is healed if the person desires it.

Finally, there is potential for the gastric band device to malfunction and breakage or leakage to occur. This is uncommon but possible. If this occurs, another procedure will be required to replace the band.

Outcomes

Studies show that, on average, patients who undergo adjustable gastric banding sustain a loss of 45–75 percent of their excess weight after two years.[8] One long-term study following patients from a single bariatric surgery center 15 years after their procedure found a sustained excess weight loss of

47 percent.[9] We have found similar results at our program in NYULMC.[10]

Which Is Right for Me?

Once you and your doctor have opted to pursue bariatric surgery, deciding which procedure is best is also a joint decision. I may think that the patient will do best with the band, but if the patient is not convinced or is unable to do the follow up, then I am not going to tell them that the band is right for them. There has to be a partnership, and it is very individual for each patient. Some people may be fearful of more invasive surgeries such as gastric bypass or sleeve gastrectomy, even though on the face of it they would be better candidates for these operations than the band.

Adjustable gastric banding is the safest and least invasive bariatric operation and is typically better for patients who don't have as much weight to lose (usually a BMI under 50). It is certainly not impossible to lose 150–200 pounds with a gastric band, but those who do are highly motivated and truly use the band as a tool rather than a crutch. If you choose a band, you must come back for regular, monthly follow-up appointments; otherwise, you will not lose weight.

The amount of weight a patient wants or needs to lose is a major consideration in the operation we choose. Closely related to that is what obesity-related health complications they are currently experiencing. If someone has type 2 diabetes and is on insulin, we would strongly encourage them to pursue the gastric bypass because of all the research we have on the success of the procedure in normalizing blood sugar levels. But, if someone just wants to lose 50–60 pounds to normalize their blood pressure and improve their mobility, then gastric banding might be preferable.

On average, the band will give you 20 pounds less weight loss than the other two operations. So, if a patient accepts that, then we are fine. But, if someone needs to lose 120 pounds in eight months because their orthopedic surgeon won't do a knee replacement at their current weight, then a better choice might be gastric bypass or a sleeve gastrectomy. The bottom line is that doctor and patient must have a full discussion about clinical goals, life after surgery, and personal preferences to arrive at a decision that's right for the individual.

Healthy Eating after Bariatric Surgery

If you choose to have bariatric surgery, no matter what procedure you have, your eating habits must necessarily change. You'll eat less, and you'll eat more slowly. It takes about 20 seconds for a piece of food to go from your mouth into your stomach, so this is how long you will need to wait between bites, after swallowing and before taking the next mouthful. This also allows you to chew thoroughly, which will help ease the passage of food through your altered digestive system.

If you eat faster than your food can travel, you will throw it back up. That's a behavioral change that you have to accept and make after surgery. If you don't, you get constant vomiting. And, if someone has a gastric band, vomiting can lead to the stomach pushing itself up through the band and the band sliding down the stomach, causing a band slippage, where it loses its effectiveness. Chronic vomiting or regurgitation is also not healthy for you.

The new sense of fullness signals that bariatric surgery creates for you will help regulate your portion sizes. You'll feel full after one slice of pizza and not want to eat the entire pie. Most people will find that a half of a normal serving size of most foods is sufficient to fill them up. There is no special liquid diet required after the first month of surgery; you eat real, healthy foods—just smaller portions consumed slowly.

Other eating ground rules include:

- *Avoiding liquid calories.* Liquid is the most easily digested item both before and after surgery, and if you continue to drink regular soda, flavored milk, fruit juice, and other sugary options, you will not lose or will regain weight.
- *Eating protein first.* Protein will fill you up and it's good for you. This is particularly important with gastric bypass, since we know that people who have this operation can become protein deficient.
- *Minimizing carbohydrates.* Carbs make you hungry by raising and then lowering your blood sugar. This is called reactive hypoglycemia and is strongest after ingesting processed sugars such as bread, cereal, baked goods, and candy. Choose high-fiber, low-glycemic index carbs and have them after your protein food. If you have a gastric bypass and you eat too much sugar or starch, you may experience *dumping syndrome.* This is characterized by sweating, flushed skin, rapid heart rate, a drop in blood pressure, nausea, diarrhea, and shakiness. It typically passes in 30–45 minutes.
- *Dealing with social pressures.* It takes some emotional work to eat appropriately after surgery, too. Food is associated with appreciation and love in many cultures, and the ability to not get caught up in social pressures to overconsume is important to your postoperative success.

We've already talked about the possibility for nutritional deficiencies with some of the bariatric procedures. We do recommend that our patients take a daily multivitamin following surgery as a preventative measure. In addition, we have their blood tests checked every three months for the first year, and then annually thereafter. It's very important to check the parathyroid hormone level in patients after gastric bypass to make sure that they don't have a calcium deficiency. Parathyroid hormone signals the body to break down bone for supplementary calcium when it senses the body is not getting enough calcium from food.

In a nutshell, you have to start being a "Mindful Eater" after bariatric surgery if you want to achieve the best benefits and the least negative side effects. If you treat surgery as "magic" and do not pay attention to what it is doing for you, then you will either not lose weight or regain weight you have lost, or you may develop serious medical problems from low vitamin or protein levels.

References

1. Buchwald H, et al. Bariatric surgery: A systematic review and meta-analysis. *JAMA*. 2014; 292(12): 1724–37.
2. Adams TD, et al. Long-term mortality after gastric bypass surgery. *N Engl J Med*. 2007 Aug 23; 357(8): 753–61.
3. Alvarez-Leite JI. Nutrient deficiencies secondary to bariatric surgery. *Curr Opin Clin Nutr Metab Care*. 2004 Sep; 7(5): 569–75. Review.
4. Andrews RA, Lim RB. Surgical management of severe obesity. In: *UpToDate*, Jones, D and Pi-Sunyar, FX (Eds), UpToDate, Waltham, MA. Accessed on July 27, 2014.
5. Buchwald H, Avidor Y, Braunwald E, et al. Bariatric surgery: A systematic review and meta-analysis. *JAMA* 2004; 292: 1724.
6. Heber D, et al. Endocrine and nutritional management of the post-bariatric surgery patient: An Endocrine Society clinical practice guideline. *J Clin Endocrin Metab*. 2010; 95(11): 4823–4843.
7. Andrews RA, Lim RB. Surgical management of severe obesity. In: *UpToDate*, Jones, D and Pi-Sunyar, FX (Eds), UpToDate, Waltham, MA. Accessed on July 27, 2014.

8. Andrews RA, Lim RB. Surgical management of severe obesity. In: *UpToDate*, Jones, D and Pi-Sunyar, FX (Eds), UpToDate, Waltham, MA. Accessed on July 27, 2014.

9. O'Brien PE, MacDonald L, Anderson M, Brennan L, Brown WA. Long-term outcomes after bariatric surgery: Fifteen-year follow-up of adjustable gastric banding and a systematic review of the bariatric surgical literature. *Ann Surg.* 2013 Jan; 257(1): 87–94. doi: 10.1097/SLA.0b013e31827b6c02. Review.

10. Carelli AM, Youn HA, Kurian MS, Ren CJ, Fielding GA. Safety of the laparoscopic adjustable gastric band: 7-year data from a U.S. center of excellence. *Surg Endosc.* 2010 Aug; 24(8): 1819–23.

Tips for Talking to Your Doctor

What is the follow-up routine for the surgery I've chosen?

_____

_____

_____

_____

_____

Should I see a dietitian? What will eating be like after surgery?

_____

_____

_____

_____

_____

How much weight should I expect to lose?

_____

_____

_____

_____

_____

_____

CHAPTER 10

Finding Answers with Your Doctor

Pete's Story

Pete is a 45-year-old man who has been suffering from chronic leg and back pain for the past six months. Pete was always of average weight for his 5'8" frame, but when his kids were born in his late thirties he stopped going to the gym regularly and put on 10 unwanted pounds. His BMI was still considered in the normal range, however, until now. Pete recently gained 15 pounds and is now overweight.

The pain has caused him to stop exercising completely, and he also admits to feeling down about his health and eating a lot more as a comfort measure. As a result, he has gained 15 additional pounds and his pain level is now increasing. He's always tired and irritable, and his wife has finally convinced him to come in and get checked out.

Pete's medical history reveals he was diagnosed with a herniated disc a few years ago, so the pain he is experiencing is likely related sciatica. Chronic pain can be a significant driver in weight gain, so I give Pete a thorough assessment and we develop a treatment plan together.

My Approach

There's a new imperative and paradigm shift that has occurred in this country. The National Heart, Lung, and Blood Institute

(NHLBI) has developed new guidelines with reference to obesity.[1] Doctors need to take the lead on diagnosing weight problems and treat them at every visit the way they would any other chronic disease. It's understandable why doctors have been reluctant to fill this role in the past. This disease is tough; it's easier to cure patients of certain malignancies than it is to effectively treat obesity.

Sometimes, doctors can get frustrated when a significantly overweight patient comes in and says they're tired, or they're having back pain, or they're having reflux, or their blood pressure is high. Although it's clear that their obesity is a contributing factor, it's how a doctor verbalizes this and empathizes with the patient that will make a difference in working toward change. It's important to draw the cause and effect line between weight and the health problem to the patient, while at the same time explaining the biological drivers that are contributing to the weight problem. And, it's critical to explore together what barriers the patient may be facing in their efforts to achieve weight loss and health gain, and how they can get past them.

The first challenge is simply broaching the subject with patients. If a patient comes in for an unrelated medical issue (e.g., a urinary tract infection, a migraine), the doctor needs to have the skill to invite the patient to return in the future for a discussion on weight. And that invitation needs to be made tactfully. We should ask your permission to discuss body weight issues, in the context of helping to improve your overall wellness.

What Are Our Goals?

My goal, and the goal of all physicians, is to improve the quality of people's lives, reduce suffering, and prevent and treat illnesses. That should be the lens through which we view the management of obesity. It is a fundamental shift in the treatment of obesity that we don't focus on weight, but instead focus on improving overall health and quality of life of the patient. Our goal is not to achieve an ideal body weight, but to reduce weight to the point where it will have a positive impact on your health. Although some would consider this goal modest, as a physician I consider it very significant. A 5–10 percent reduction in weight can make a tremendous difference in wellness, and achieving it is a success from my viewpoint.

Even this "modest" weight loss can be challenging to achieve and sustain. Both doctor and patient should have an understanding of the complexity and difficulty of keeping weight off long-term. Because obesity is a chronic illness, there will be times when the disease becomes more active and weight maintenance is more challenging, and patients need to be made aware of that so they don't get too frustrated or discouraged.

It's important that doctor and patient both measure success by determining whether or not improvements are made in physical, mental, and metabolic measures. Do their knees feel better? Has their blood pressure gone down? Are they sleeping better and feeling more energetic? Are their blood sugar and cholesterol values improving? Together, we look for measurable parameters that will help determine whether we are really making progress. Progress is made and progress is measured. Again, it's more than simply weight.

Finally, perhaps the most important thing for both doctor and patient to remember is that when it comes to the management of obesity, one size does not fit all. What works for one patient may not work for another patient. Doctors need to educate themselves about the wide variety of treatment options available today, including drugs and surgery. And patients need to realize that the surgery that helped their coworker drop 100 pounds, or the diet plan that their neighbor swears by, may not necessarily be right for them. Treating overweight and obesity requires a customized approach. And the first step to that is having a comprehensive assessment with your doctor.

The Physical Assessment

The physical assessment is similar to a wellness physical, in that we want to get an idea of your current overall state of health, plus any factors that put you at risk for health conditions. A physical assessment should include:

- *Body composition measurements.* Weight, BMI, body fat percentage, and waist circumference can help us establish your level of fitness and risk for health issues (see chapter 6 for a description of these tests). It also gives us a baseline against which to measure your future progress.
- *Lab tests.* A complete blood count (CBC) can provide a good look at your current state of health. We also look at cholesterol and hemoglobin A1C (long-term blood sugar) levels, as we know these are two markers on which weight can have a negative influence. Additional blood and urine tests may be ordered based on your family and health history.
- *Physical exam.* Taking blood pressure; listening to the heart and lungs; checking reflexes; checking ears, nose, and throat; and doing a basic examination of the body can help diagnose health issues.
- *Medications.* Drugs can be a barrier to success. Beta blockers, antipsychotics, antidepressants, and diabetes drugs may be contributing to weight gain or related

health issues. It's important to have a comprehensive list of prescription and over-the-counter medicines.

• *Family history.* Finding out if there is a history of weight problems in the family may point to a genetic predisposition.

• *Health history.* If you don't have a long history with your doctor, it's helpful to fill them in on any surgeries, major illnesses, or injuries that have occurred in your life.

The Lifestyle Assessment

After a full physical assessment and history, it's important to find out what life circumstances and choices might be influencing the patient's health. The lifestyle assessment is just as important as the physical assessment in determining a realistic plan of action for weight management.

The overwhelming majority of people I see with weight-related health problems have a past history of trying to lose weight. As part of the assessment, your doctor should get a history about your past experiences. Is weight gain recent or has it been a lifelong problem? When did it start? Have you tried to lose weight in the past? If so, how and were you successful? Did something happen in your life that you think contributed to the weight gain?

Life disruption, or what I call "chaos," is a critical driver of weight gain. Anything that causes chaos in your life, good or bad, can trigger weight gain. Moving, a new job, starting school, graduating, births, deaths, marriage, divorce—all take an emotional toll and the physical impact of this chaos is associated with biological changes that can impact hunger and the sense of fullness. This will affect weight and how we treat it. I always ask my patients about recent chaos in their life that could be impacting their health. I encourage you to share this information with your doctor, as it may influence the treatment plan.

Other lifestyle issues you should discuss with your doctor include:

- **Home responsibilities.** People caring for an elderly parent or small children may face additional stress or financial or time constraints.
- **Occupation and schedule.** Work schedules can interfere with appropriate sleep, exercise, and eating right.
- **Socioeconomics.** Does a lack of financial resources promote unhealthy eating and other behaviors? Do you live in an area where outside exercise isn't possible due to safety issues?

Choosing the Right Tools

Once this assessment is complete, we can use this information to determine a treatment path (see Table 3). I work with my patients to create parameters. What is our goal in the first month? In the first three months? It's important to be flexible. Lives change, and chaos comes out of nowhere. Once you have made the commitment to the hard work of behavior and lifestyle change, we want to set realistic weight loss goals that will pay off in health benefits.

So, how much weight will you need to lose to make meaningful changes in your blood pressure, cholesterol levels, blood sugar levels, sleep apnea, joint and back pain, or other health issues?

If your BMI is 25 or over, the NHLBI recommends an initial weight loss goal of 10 percent of body weight within six months. This allows for weight loss of one to two pounds a

Table 3. Selecting Treatment Guidelines

Treatment	BMI Category				
	25–26.9	27–29.9	30–34.9	35–39.9	≥40
Diet, physical activity & behavioral therapy	With comorbidities	With comorbidities	+	+	+
Pharmacotherapy* (drug)		With comorbidities	+	+	+
Surgery				With comorbidities	+

The + represents the use of indicated treatment regardless of comorbidities.
*Consider pharmacotherapy only if a patient has not lost 1 pound per week after 6 months of combined lifestyle therapy.
Source: Adapted from Practical guide to the identification, evaluation and treatment of overweight and obesity in adults. National Institutes of Health; National Heart, Lung and Blood Institute; North American Association for the Study of Obesity. October 2000.

week, depending on your starting BMI. The joint obesity guidelines issued by the American Heart Association, American College of Cardiology, and the Obesity Society suggest a slightly different goal of 5–10 percent weight loss within six months. If health goals aren't achieved with that loss, additional goals can be set.

But again, one size does not fit all. We know that sustained weight loss of as little as 3–5 percent of body weight can produce clinically meaningful reductions in triglycerides, blood sugar, and type 2 diabetes risk.[2] It's possible that a lower goal may give you significant health benefits. And, it's also possible that some weight-related health conditions may require more than a 10 percent weight reduction to resolve or show improvement.

Lifestyle is the most critical component to treatment. This

is where you, the patient, are really taking control. First is a shift in how you think about food. From this point forward, diet must be thought of as a lifelong way of healthy eating, not a short-term restrictive plan to drop weight. Your doctor can provide a referral to a registered dietitian, who can help you develop a better understanding of food as a nutrient and suggest meal plans based on your recommended calorie intake.

Start putting premium fuel in your body—plenty of fruits, vegetables, fiber, and lean protein. A modest reduction in portions and in total calories, especially carbohydrates, is important. But, it is important not to restrict calories too dramatically; a drop of about 500 calories daily is recommended. Your physician, or a registered dietitian, can recommend an appropriate daily calorie level based on your height, weight, activity level, and weight loss goals. Keeping track of your food intake with a food diary or app is important in staying on top of both calories and the nutrient value of your food.

Your second essential tool is activity. Again, this is working exercise into your everyday life, with a focus on long-term health, not a short-term quick weight loss. Exercise is the only way to increase your level of cardiorespiratory fitness, which is key to heart and metabolic health; nutrition alone won't do this (see chapter 6 for more information on cardiorespiratory fitness). And, physical activity independent of calorie reduction can produce a 2–3 percent decrease in body weight.

To increase your energy burn, the exercise has to be modest to moderate intensity. You may need some training, and you may need a medical clearance before you start working out. If you have several risk factors for heart disease and you are currently inactive, an exercise stress test might be recommended to ensure that you exercise at a level that is safe for your heart. That's why the physician is such an important component; they need to guide you from a medical point of view for the safety of your exercise program.

It's very important for you and your doctor to talk about barriers to exercise. If you work long hours or travel a lot for work, you may have trouble working in a regular gym routine. Even the busiest people can find some time to get active during the day; it just may take some creativity to work it in. And it doesn't have to be done "all at once." You may start by committing to a brisk lunchtime walk or do something as simple as taking the stairs instead of the elevator to your office. An exercise physiologist or a trainer may be helpful in putting some structure around your exercise plans, and your doctor can refer you to these resources.

I also encourage my patients to take advantage of the growing number of devices available that can monitor your activity during the day. These are great for holding yourself accountable to daily activity and for motivating yourself toward new goals. They range from simple step counters to more sophisticated activity and sleep trackers that sync with your wireless device. And they don't have to be expensive; you can pick up a no-frills clip-on pedometer for less than $10.

Beyond lifestyle change, we do have other weight-management tools at our disposal. For those who are obese with comorbidities (obesity-related health problems) and who have tried and failed to achieve sustained weight loss with lifestyle change, drug therapy or bariatric surgery may be appropriate.

A Team Effort

Some weight-related complications need extra care from a specialist. People with diabetes may benefit from an appointment with an endocrinologist. Others may need to see a urologist, or a gynecologist, or an orthopedist, depending on their issues. And, because depression is so common in people who are overweight or obese, a psychiatrist or therapist may be an important member of the team.

It's critical for your doctor to pull other treating physicians into the conversation, especially if they are prescribing drugs that may be contributing to weight gain. If I have a patient who is on an antidepressant that is known to cause weight gain, and he's already struggling with hypertension and pre-diabetes, I would have a conversation with his consulting psychiatrist about other drug options for him.

Weight loss for health gain is hard work, for both the doctor and especially the patient. And this is why your readiness for change is so important. Most of the control is in your hands; there is no magic pill or surgical treatment that will work without your dedication to healthy lifestyle changes. While your doctor can guide you, make suggestions, and track your progress, only you can make the life changes critical to success.

So, make sure you are open with your doctor about past challenges and current barriers, and ask questions if you don't understand the goals he/she is suggesting or the steps to take to get there. Ask for referrals to nutrition and exercise specialists if you need additional guidance. Use the questions in this book to inform your conversations with your doctor.

Pete, Revisited

Pete feels strongly, and I agree, that losing this recent 15-pound weight gain will probably relieve the pain significantly. Our assessment reveals that Pete's dietary patterns at mealtime are actually fairly healthy; his issues come up when he starts feeling physically and mentally bad and binges on snack foods to self-medicate. It's clear that exercise is the missing component in his life.

The immediate barrier to exercise is the pain he's experiencing. Pete has had a previous bad reaction to cortisone injections, so instead I put him on a regimen of anti-inflammatory drugs and physical therapy to provide some relief, improve his sleep, and get him moving again. During our assessment Pete mentions he enjoys swimming, so I suggest he spend a few mornings a week doing laps at his local YMCA, along with some simple strength training exercises.

I also refer Pete to a psychologist because of a past history of depression that appears to have resurfaced. I follow up with the psychologist to advise him of our weight loss goal so that if he and Pete decide on a trial of medication, they can choose one that doesn't promote weight gain.

Four months later, Pete comes in for a follow up. He has lost 10 pounds on the scale, but more importantly, he is pain free and his mood is significantly better. He reports swimming an hour in the morning most days of the week and having much greater energy. And it's clear he's gained some muscle tone from his strength training routine. Pete sets another goal of 10–15 pounds to achieve in the next six months. I caution him that weight loss does get harder after the first six months of a program, and not to get discouraged if he doesn't get there as long as he is feeling great both physically and mentally.

References

1. *Practical guide to the identification, evaluation and treatment of overweight and obesity in adults.* National Institutes of Health; National Heart, Lung and Blood Institute; North American Association for the Study of Obesity. October 2000.
2. Mechanick JI, Youdim A, Jones DB, et al. American Association of Clinical Endocrinologists, Obesity Society, American Society for Metabolic & Bariatric Surgery. Clinical practice guidelines for the perioperative nutritional, metabolic, and nonsurgical support of the bariatric surgery patient—2013 update: cosponsored by American Association of Clinical Endocrinologists, the Obesity Society, and American Society for Metabolic & Bariatric Surgery. *Endocr Pract.* 2013 Mar–Apr; 19(2): 337–72.

Tips for Talking to Your Doctor

Should I see a specialist for my diabetes, joint pain, or other health conditions?

_____

_____

_____

_____

Do I need an exercise stress test before I start working out?

_____

_____

_____

_____

What is a realistic goal for a six-month weight loss, and by what health measurements will we confirm success?

_____

_____

_____

_____

Balance for Life

Personalized Medicine

I strongly believe there has to be a personalized approach to all aspects of weight management. Although they may have exactly the same BMI and a similar health history, a woman who has two small children and works from home may have very different needs from the woman who has to travel 8–10 days a month for her job. It's not just about giving everybody the same diet, the same drugs, the same exercise program, and that's probably why commercial diet programs are rarely a successful solution for people struggling with weight loss. That's part of the art of medicine and why you need a physician with whom to work.

What you're seeing is that one size does not fit all. What may work for one individual may not be successful for others because of the barriers outlined in this book. Some of the patient stories in this book may resonate with you and give you ideas to talk about with your doctor. Then together, you can tailor a program that works for you.

The Sleep-Weight Connection

Everyone knows what sleep is, but most people don't understand the words *circadian rhythm*. Humans have a certain biological rhythm governed by an internal 24-hour clock. The circadian rhythm regulates many things, from hormone release to body temperature, but a primary task is regulating wakefulness during the daytime and sleepiness at night. As we start to play with Mother Nature by changing our normal sleep-wakefulness pattern, we create disorganization or disregulation in our circadian rhythms. And it's not just the length of sleep, but also the quality and timing of that sleep that are important to your metabolic health. One of the consequences of the circadian disruption may be an increased risk of obesity, diabetes, heart disease, depression, and cancer.[1, 2, 3, 4, 5]

We also know sleep deprivation promotes excessive

caloric and fat intake, likely due to increases in ghrelin production (which makes us hungry and can alter our food preferences) and decreases in leptin, the "fullness" hormone.[6] When we get chronically sleepy, we get hungry, and we are also less likely to have the energy to go and burn off those extra calories through activity.[7]

Work, social demands, and other commitments keep everyone busy, and sleep is often the first thing we sacrifice to find the time to "do it all." An occasional late night won't damage your health, but if it becomes a chronic pattern, it's important to reevaluate your priorities and make the time for regular, restful sleep.

Of course, circumstances may prevent you from proper sleep hygiene—for example, if you have an infant at home (fortunately, your child's circadian rhythms will soon settle into a pattern more consistent with your adult need for sleep). More difficult to address are the needs of the 15 million Americans working irregular schedules—from night shifts to rotating shifts or extended hours. Fortunately, there are ways to nudge our circadian phases into adapting to our schedule by manipulating zeitgebers.

A *zeitgeber* is an environmental cue that helps synchronize our circadian clock. Light is one of the most critical ones. Our circadian rhythms are controlled by the suprachiasmatic nucleus (SCN), an area in the hypothalamus of the brain. When the SCN senses light or dark signals from our eyes, it triggers chemical messengers to either wake us up or make us tired.[8] In the presence of light, the SCN sends signals to raise body temperature and release cortisol, and in darkness, it lowers body temperature and stimulates melatonin production by the pineal gland.

Overnight shift workers can bypass some of the ill health effects of circadian disruption by using light to their advantage to reprogram their circadian phases. Dark sunglasses should be worn on the commute home, and sleep should be scheduled immediately following the overnight shift. The sleep environment should be kept as dark as possible with blackout curtains. Conversely, exposure to bright light during waking and working hours is important in shifting the circadian sleep cycle.[9]

In addition to manipulating light, melatonin supplementation taken before sleep may help improve the length and quality of sleep in shift workers trying to adjust their circadian phases. However, there is conflicting research on its effectiveness for this purpose and for treating insomnia. More large-scale studies are needed to determine if melatonin supplements are helpful; however, given that the supplement carries a low risk of side effects, there is probably no harm in trying it. But, as with any supplement, you should talk to your doctor before taking melatonin.

Here are a few simple measures everyone can take to promote better sleep and better metabolic health.

- ***Turn off the lights and the smartphones.*** Again, light—even electronic screen lights—can trigger a cascade of hormones that interfere with sleep. A dark sleep environment, without glowing smartphones or other screens to trigger wakefulness, is important.

- ***Keep a schedule.*** If, due to work or other circumstances, you must sleep outside what your circadian clock deems normal, be consistent. Your body will adapt better if sleep comes at the same time each day. And nightshift workers should try to plan sleep within 1–2 hours after the end of work.

- ***Skip late-night snacks.*** If you have diabetes or prediabetes, late-night eating can elevate blood sugars more than daytime eating and can make blood glucose levels harder to manage the next morning.[10, 11]

- *Catch up when you can.* If you've had a period of poor sleep due to vacation, illness, or other temporary chaos in your life, the important thing is to recover and return to a consistent pattern of 7–9 hours of sleep each evening. We know that the effects of sleep deprivation seem to be reversible after a period of sufficient sleep during normal hours.

How to Break the Stress Cycle

Two of the most fundamental and primary drivers for weight gain are stress and chaos. Almost universally, people who have gained 15 or 20 pounds over a six-month to one-year period have had a very chaotic period in their lives. Whether it's a change in job, having a child, going to school or college, graduate school, law school, getting married or divorced, financial reversals, or any other life change, both good and bad stress can cause weight gain.

We know that daily exposure to stress can cause weight gain; one study of breast cancer patients found that daily stress exposure resulted in metabolic changes that could result in an 11-pound weight gain each year.[12] Chronic stress promotes visceral fat accumulation, increases appetite, and enhances a preference for those calorie-dense comfort foods that are high in fat and/or sugar and promote weight gain.[13]

Because I know chaos and resulting stress contribute to weight gain, I tell people before the occurrence of a known life change that they are going to be at risk for gaining weight. It's important to initiate a program before they gain the weight and encourage a certain activity level and nutrient intake so they don't gain more than five pounds. It's a risk management approach. We know it's going to happen, but we can blunt the response and reduce the impact.

It's also important to encourage outlets for stress management. In addition to blunting weight gain, exercise is a proven stress buster. So are meditation, guided imagery, and simply engaging in a hobby or activity you enjoy (e.g., gardening, dancing). Make time for an activity that relaxes you and/or makes you feel good. This is important not just in times of chaos, but as part of a holistic healthy lifestyle.

Meals, Movement, and More

One of my favorite cities on the planet to visit is Venice, Italy. Despite the abundance of restaurants there, I rarely see an overweight Venetian. In fact, the adult obesity rate in Italy is far lower than in America. Why? I'm sure the predominant way of eating—the Mediterranean diet—has something to do with it. It's chock full of vegetables, fruits, nuts, and whole grains instead of processed foods; olive oil instead of butter; herbs and spices instead of salt; and fish and poultry instead of red meat. And studies have shown that it can be a powerful tool in long-term weight management and promoting heart health.[14, 15]

In addition to these healthy eating habits, Venetians spend a lot of time being physically active. Venice is built on more than 100 small islands connected by canals and bridges, so to get anywhere you either float or walk. With more than 400 footbridges threading through the city and breathtaking views everywhere, it's a pedestrian's paradise. Between all this exercise and the sustained healthy diet, Venetians appear to be exceedingly fit. Of course, we can't all move to Venice, but I think there is something Americans can learn from this cultural perspective.

As we've said throughout this book, lifestyle change for

weight management and health is not a short-term fix—it's a lifetime goal. And that goal is to make positive changes around food and exercise part of the fabric of your everyday life, just like a Venetian.

It bears repeating that you should emphasize the nutrient value of the foods you eat and think in terms of enhancing and improving it instead of thinking only in terms of calorie restriction. This goes not just for weight loss and short-term health benefits, but for lifetime wellness.

There are many "systems of eating" like the Mediterranean diet that can be successful. There is no single "right" way to eat well, but there are some basic rules to follow based on nutrition research. It makes sense to eat whole foods (unprocessed), fruits, vegetables, lean protein, and plenty of fiber in your diet. Choose low-glycemic carbohydrates, which are generally those with the most fiber (e.g., cruciferous vegetables, berries, whole grains). You may want to lower the amount of saturated fat you eat.[16]

If you are vegan or vegetarian, you can still make these changes. But keep in mind that veganism or vegetarianism does not necessarily make you achieve an ideal weight. You still need a mix of nutrients, including protein, in your diet. You still need to think in terms of the long-term overall nutrient value of the foods you are taking in. If you are struggling with food choices, vegan or otherwise, please see a registered dietitian for help. They are trained to work with you to create an individual meal plan based on your caloric needs, lifestyle, and food preferences.

The other essential ingredient for maintaining your weight and wellness long term is exercise. If you aren't increasing your level of cardiovascular fitness through regular aerobic and strength training exercise, you are shortening your life.[17] It's that simple. Again, if you need help, ask for it. A trainer or an exercise physiologist can help you develop a routine that works for your skill level and lifestyle.

The best way to ensure you keep moving is to do something you enjoy. Walking is great for the Venetians, but perhaps it's not for you. If you hate the treadmill, get off of it. From dancing to roller skating, there are hundreds of ways to exercise. Find a few you like and make exercise a passion, not a chore.

Supplements for Weight Management

Most nutrients should come from the foods we eat. But, for those we don't get (or don't get enough of) in food, supplements may be helpful. People who go on restrictive diets that compromise nutrition intake can probably benefit most from supplements. But, understand that supplements are just an additional tool for wellness, not a panacea. When I recommend a supplement, it's for the purpose of providing nutrients to promote good health, not for fueling weight loss. That's why I favor supplements such as omega-3s, vitamin D, and flavonoids. Flavonoids are plant-based chemicals (phytochemicals) that have antioxidant, anticancer, anti-inflammatory, antiviral, and antibacterial properties.[18] Dietary sources of these disease-fighting substances include green tea, dark chocolate, red wine, and myriad fruits and vegetables.

Probiotics and prebiotics are two supplements that do hold some promise to digestive and metabolic health and weight management. Early studies show that microbiota in your gut may play a role in the development of metabolic disease, and that both pre- and probiotics may help promote gut health and modulate the metabolic response.[19] More studies are needed to establish this link.

It's important to realize that supplements are not regulated as stringently as prescription and over-the-counter drugs. They come in a variety of potencies and quality levels; if you are interested in trying a supplement, please ask your doctor about what's appropriate for you and get a recommendation for dosage and brand.

It Takes a Village

As we said at the beginning of this book, it will take a societal effort to tackle the problem of obesity in America. We need to move away from blame to come up with a solution, and it will take every sector of society to contribute toward lowering the obesity rate and raising the level of health in this country.

Government
We need to teach nutrition and healthy eating in the schools as early as the kids can appreciate it, and improve federal food labeling guidelines so that it's easier for Americans to make smarter food choices.

Family and Friends
Social support makes a huge difference; if you feel emotionally supported in pursuing healthy behaviors, it's easier to stick with them. Pursue wellness as a family, not only for yourself but for your children and grandchildren. Overweight parents often have overweight kids, so breaking the cycle is important.

Healthcare
In declaring obesity a chronic disease state, the medical community has made a huge step toward destigmatizing and properly treating obesity and excess weight. We need to keep moving in that direction. One of my colleagues recently went for an internal medicine board review, which is what an internist

must do to retain their credentials. During the board review course there was a new focus on the role of internists and managing obesity as a chronic disease, along with a review of new treatment options. That is a huge and exciting step in the right direction. I've always believed that a primary care doctor must manage obesity in their practice; otherwise, they are just using Band-Aids to treat the symptoms.

Society

Obesity remains very much stigmatized in this country. Estimates show that the prevalence of weight discrimination has actually increased by 66 percent in the past decade and is now comparable to rates of racial discrimination in America. There is a good amount of evidence that this stigmatization actually perpetuates the cycle of weight gain and obesity and also takes a serious toll on psychological health.[20] You have now seen the overwhelming evidence that weight is not a will-power issue, but a serious health problem driven by complex biological, neurological, and environmental factors. We can all do our part in reversing weight stigma and discrimination by challenging media campaigns and other public and private conversations that marginalize the overweight. Speak up ... your voice can make a difference.

You

Most importantly, you need to take personal responsibility for improving your health. Only you can exercise, eat right, and sleep enough. My goal is to ultimately do less for you, the patient. I want to subtract medications for hypertension and high cholesterol as your weight drops and your fitness level improves. The more you do for yourself, the less I need to intervene. Your doctor is there to coach you and give you tools, but only you can play the game.

What the Future Holds

This is an exciting time for the science of weight loss for wellness. Every month there is a new scientific finding or discovery that furthers our understanding and provides more information for new treatments.

We talked about some of the new obesity drugs in chapter 7. There are also new medical devices currently in clinical trials. Although these currently are not available for use in the United States (except in clinical trials), they may provide more tools for people struggling with weight and health issues

The Obalon balloon (Obalon Therapeutics) is an investigational device that has helped trial participants lose an average of 34–50 percent of excess body weight in clinical studies.[21] The device works by making patients feel full with smaller meals through the use of a gastric balloon. The deflated balloon is packaged inside of a small, dissolving capsule that is attached to a thin tube. After a patient swallows the capsule, the balloon is inflated through the tube, and the tube is then removed. Up to three balloons can be swallowed and inflated. After three months, the balloons are removed endoscopically.

The EndoBarrier (GI Dynamics) is an intestinal "liner" that is placed endoscopically in the upper colon. It creates a barrier between food and the duodenum, the area of the intestines that absorbs nutrients. In this respect, it mimics the effects of gastric bypass surgery without the surgery. In trials, the EndoBarrier has resulted in an average loss of 12–22 percent of excess weight.[22] It has also demonstrated a very positive impact on normalizing blood sugar in people with type 2 diabetes.

Summing It All Up

Achieving weight loss and wellness is not for the faint hearted. It takes a dedicated patient, a knowledgeable doctor, and a lot of hard work. You will have to break some hard habits, and depending on your situation, it may require surgery or medication to achieve better health. Yes, it's difficult, but it's also extremely satisfying when you make these life changes and start to see results—in lower blood sugar, normal blood pressure, increased energy, improved mood, less pain, better sleep, and an enhanced quality of life.

Because obesity is a chronic condition, there will occasionally be feelings of hopelessness and frustration on both parts. Weight maintenance is often harder than the initial weight loss. As you now know, it's normal for your body to rebel against your efforts, and putting pounds back on is common. Do not feel embarrassed to return to your doctor when it happens; no one will judge you or be angry with you. Medication may need to be changed, and new barriers to weight loss may need to be addressed. Remember, this is a marathon, not a sprint, and your doctor is there to help you stay on track. Above all, don't give up. The stakes—your health, your happiness, and your lifespan—are just too high. It's time for ALL of us to get serious about healthy weight management for life.

This is the dawn of a new era for everyone struggling with weight-related health problems. We have more treatment tools than ever before and an evolving body of scientific research that is opening up new possibilities for the future. It's an exciting time for both healthcare professionals and patients. I wish you well in your journey toward better health.

Sam, Revisited

Sam's biggest barrier is his job, but it's also the barrier least likely to change. He enjoys what he does for a living, and his salary gives him a comfortable living. So, we look at what we can do to get past this by customizing our own approach.

We put Sam on a trial of Belviq to help suppress his appetite. I explain that he should anticipate a modest weight loss of at least 5 percent over the next 12 weeks, but that amount is significant enough to have a positive impact on his health. The company Sam works for is opening an on-site employee gym the next month, and he thinks this access is just what he needs to keep up his exercise routine. We also discuss what time is optimal to exercise and eat depending on his shift. I send him to a registered dietitian to come up with an eating plan that works for his crazy schedule. She alerts him to a service that delivers his groceries by appointment for a nominal fee, and they come up with a variety of low-effort meals that Sam can eat at home and on the job.

Sam initially loses 40 pounds, which puts him solidly at a "normal" BMI and past his goal of 25 pounds. But, one year later, he had regained eight pounds. Because we'd talked about the probability of weight regain, and Sam had kept up on his gym routine and healthy nutrition, this didn't deter him. His latest blood work shows that his cholesterol and A1C levels have returned to the normal target range.

References

1. Grandner MA, Jackson NJ, Pak VM, Gehrman PR. Sleep disturbance is associated with cardiovascular and metabolic disorders. *J Sleep Res.* 2012 Aug; 21(4): 427–33.
2. Nakata A. Work hours, sleep sufficiency, and prevalence of depression among full-time employees: A community-based cross-sectional study. *J Clin Psychiatry.* 2011 May; 72(5): 605–14.
3. Nakata A, Irie M, Takahashi M. Association of general fatigue with cellular immune indicators among healthy white-collar employees. *J Occup Environ Med.* 2011. Sep; 53(9): 1078–86.
4. Violanti JM, Burchfiel CM, Hartley TA, et al. Atypical work hours and metabolic syndrome among police officers. *Arch Environ Occup Health.* 2009; 64(3): 194–201.
5. Sheikh-Ali M, Maharaj J. Circadian clock desynchronisation and metabolic syndrome. *Postgrad Med J.* 2014 Aug; 90(1066): 461–466. doi: 10.1136/postgradmedj-2013-132366. Epub 2014 Jun 23. Review.
6. Taheri S, Lin L, Austin D, Young T, Mignot E. Short sleep duration is associated with reduced leptin, elevated ghrelin, and increased body mass index. *PLoS Med.* 2004 Dec; 1(3): e62.
7. Spaeth AM, Dinges DF, Goel N. Effects of experimental sleep restriction on weight gain, caloric intake, and meal timing in healthy adults. *Sleep.* 2013; 36(7): 981–990.
8. Fonken LK, Nelson RJ. The effects of light at night on circadian clocks and metabolism. *Endocr Rev.* 2014 Apr; 35(4): 648–70. doi: 10.1210/er.2013-1051.
9. Revell VL, Eastman CI. How to trick mother nature into letting you fly around or stay up all night. *J Biol Rhythms.* 2005 Aug; 20(4): 353–65.
10. Sato M, Nakamura K, Ogata H, et al. Acute effect of late evening meal on diurnal variation of blood glucose and energy metabolism. *Obes Res Clin Pract.* 2011 Jul–Sep; 5(3): e169–266.
11. Tsuchida Y, Hata S, Sone Y. Effects of a late supper on digestion and the absorption of dietary carbohydrates in the following morning. *J Physiol Anthropol.* 2013 May 25; 32(1): 9.
12. Kiecolt-Glaser JK, Habash DL, Fagundes CP, et al. Daily stressors, past depression, and metabolic responses to high-fat meals: A novel path to obesity. *Biol Psychiatry.* 2014 Jul 9. pii: S0006-3223(14)00385-0. doi: 10.1016/j.biopsych.2014.05.018. [Epub ahead of print] 2014 Jul 9.
13. Sominsky L, Spencer SJ. Eating behavior and stress: A pathway to obesity. *Front Psychol.* 2014 May 13; 5: 434.
14. Esposito K, Kastorini CM, Panagiotakos DB, Giugliano D. Mediterranean diet and weight loss: Meta-analysis of randomized controlled trials. *Metab Syndr Relat Disord.* 2011 Feb; 9(1): 1–12.
15. Kastorini CM, Milionis HJ, Goudevenos JA, Panagiotakos DB. Mediterranean diet and coronary heart disease: Is obesity a link?

A systematic review. *Nutr Metab Cardiovasc Dis.* 2010 Sep; 20(7): 536–51.

16. Soeliman FA, Azadbakht L. Weight loss maintenance: A review on dietary related strategies. *J Res Med Sci.* 2014 Mar; 19(3): 268–75. Review.

17. Lee CD, Blair SN, Jackson AS. Cardiorespiratory fitness, body composition, and all-cause and cardiovascular disease mortality in men. *Am J Clin Nutr.* 1999 Mar; 69(3): 373–80.

18. Kumar S, Pandey AK. Chemistry and biological activities of flavonoids: An overview. *Scientific World Journal.* 2013 Dec 29; 2013: 162750.

19. Erejuwa OO, Sulaiman SA, Ab Wahab MS. Modulation of gut microbiota in the management of metabolic disorders: The prospects and challenges. *Int J Mol Sci.* 2014 Mar 7; 15(3): 4158–88.

20. Puhl RM, Heuer CA. Obesity stigma: Important considerations for public health. *Am J Public Health.* 2010 Jun; 100(6): 1019–28.

21. Performance of the Obalon balloon in commercial use. Obalon Therapeutics. Publication LIT-1000-0038-02.

22. Patel SR, Mason J, Hakim N. The duodenal-jejunal bypass sleeve (EndoBarrier gastrointestinal liner) for weight loss and treatment of type II diabetes. *Indian J Surg.* 2012 Aug; 74(4): 275–7.

Tips for Talking to Your Doctor

Could my sleep habits be affecting my health? Could I have a sleep disorder?

_____

_____

_____

_____

_____

Should I expect to gain some of my lost weight back? If so, what's the best strategy to minimize the regain?

_____

_____

_____

_____

_____

Do you recommend that I take any dietary supplements?

_____

_____

_____

_____

Additional Resources for Health and Weight Management

A collection of useful resources to help you in your journey toward better health.

Advocacy and Support

Obesity Action Coalition
The Obesity Action Coalition (OAC) is a national nonprofit organization "dedicated to improving the lives of individuals affected by the disease of obesity." The group publishes a monthly magazine, *Your Weight Matters*, and provides a state-by-state listing of support groups and advocacy resources.
800.717.3117
www.obesityaction.org

Obesity Help
A peer support community that "is dedicated to the education, empowerment, and support of all individuals affected by obesity, along with their families, friends, employers, surgeons, and physicians."
866.957.4636
www.obesityhelp.com

The Weight-Control Information Network (WIN)
An information service of the National Institute of Diabetes and Digestive and Kidney Diseases (NIDDK), one of the National Institutes of Health. Offers educational information on obesity, physical activity, nutrition, and other weight-related issues.
www.win.niddk.nih.gov

Bariatric/Metabolic Surgery
American Society for Metabolic and Bariatric Surgery
ASMBS Patient Learning Center
Offers educational resources on different types of bariatric surgery, as well as a searchable index of bariatric surgeons in your area.
www.asmbs.org/patients

NYU Langone Weight Management Program
This facility is recognized as a "Bariatric Center of Excellence" by the American Society for Bariatric Surgery. Dr. Christine Ren-Fielding (see chapter 9) founded the program and Dr. George Fielding (see chapter 8) is a lead surgeon at the facility. Their website offers informational videos and other educational information on surgical and nonsurgical weight loss.
212.263.3166
thinforlife.med.nyu.edu

Food and Nutrition
The Academy of Nutrition and Dietetics
The professional organization for food and nutrition professionals, also offering public education resources for healthy eating. Find a registered dietitian in your area with their online database.
www.eatright.org

David Bouley
With a focus on pure ingredients and nutrition, restaurateur and chef David Bouley is known for several New York City–based eateries that feature healthy cuisine. Bouley Botanical offers collaborative health-focused lectures and multi-course dinners curated by Chef Bouley and world-renowned doctors.
www.davidbouley.com

The Goldring Center for Culinary Medicine
A collaborative effort between Tulane University School of Medicine and Johnson & Wales College of Culinary Arts, the center seeks to teach future doctors and their patients about healthy food selection and preparation. The website features a wide selection of recipes, and the center puts on special events and community cooking classes in the New Orleans area.
www.culinarymedicine.org

Wholesome Wave
Promoting affordable, accessible, and sustainable farm-to-table eating. Offers programs at farmers markets across the country that give customers a monetary incentive to spend their federal nutrition benefits for locally grown fruits and vegetables.
www.wholesomewave.org

Smart Phone Apps
Visit the websites below for more information. All apps are currently available in both Android and iOS (iPhone) versions unless otherwise noted.
www.fooducate.com
www.gomeals.com

Exercise and Fitness
Adult Fitness Test
Part of the President's Challenge, this test will help you estimate your level of aerobic fitness, strength, flexibility, and body composition.
www.adultfitnesstest.org

The American Council on Exercise (ACE)
A nonprofit organization "committed to America's health and well-being," ACE offers certification for fitness professionals and an extensive online library of exercise and workout videos for people at all levels of fitness, from beginners to pros.
888.825.3636
www.acefitness.org

Presidential Active Lifestyle Award (PALA+)
Be physically active every day for 6–8 weeks and earn this award sponsored by the President's Council on Fitness, Sports & Nutrition. The website provides plenty of ideas for physical activity.
www.presidentschallenge.org

Tracking Devices
Activity trackers are great tools to keep track of your daily activity and motivate you toward new goals. Following is a list of manufacturer websites to find out more information.
Fitbit—www.fitbit.com
Garmin Vivofit—sites.garmin.com/vivo/
Jawbone Up—www.jawbone.com
Misfit Shine—www.misfit.com
Polar Loop—www.polarloop.com
Samsung Gearfit—www.samsung.com/GearFit

Smart Phone Apps
Smart phone apps can help track your daily activity and share the information with people you choose in your social network. Visit the websites below for more information. All apps are currently available in both Android and iOS (iPhone) versions unless otherwise noted.
www.mapmyfitness.com
www.myfitnesspal.com

Sleep Hygiene

National Sleep Foundation
Get tools and tips for better sleep, information on weight-related sleep issues (e.g., sleep apnea, shift work disorder), and find a sleep healthcare professional in your area.
www.sleepfoundation.org

Stress Management

Headspace
A free, science-based meditation program created by author, speaker, and ordained Buddhist monk Andy Puddicombe. Headspace also has an associated free app you can download to your smartphone.
www.headspace.com

American Heart Association Stress Management Center
The AHA offers tools and tips to recognize emotional and
physical stress and lower stress levels.
www.heart.org/stress

Glossary

Definitions of terms and concepts associated with the new obesity science.

Adipocyte. The fat cell. Also known as a lipocyte.

Adipokines. Substances released by fat tissue that help regulate a whole range of metabolic processes, including hunger, inflammation, blood pressure regulation, and clotting of the blood.

Adiponectin. An *adipokine* that helps regulate glucose levels by increasing insulin sensitivity and breaking down free fatty acids.

Adjustable gastric banding. Also known by the trade name Lap-Band®. This bariatric procedure involves placing an adjustable silicone band around the top of the stomach. The band is then tightened periodically to place pressure on the vagus nerve, which suppresses appetite.

Angry fat. A term used to describe fat cells when they become stressed. Angry fat promotes inflammation by producing *cytokines* and increasing circulating *free fatty acids*.

Bariatric surgery. A surgical procedure that either restricts the size of the stomach or creates changes in the digestive tract that prevent absorption of nutrients and calories. Bariatric surgery is sometimes called metabolic surgery.

Beige fat. A type of fat cell that has more mitochondria than *white fat* but fewer than *brown fat*. Mitochondria burn glucose and fat.

Body fat percentage. The percentage of fat mass in your body versus your total body mass. Women should have a body fat percentage of 31 percent or less, and men should be at 25 percent or less.

Body mass index (BMI). A measure of body fatness calculated from a person's height and weight. It is used to screen adults and children for potential weight problems and is used in population studies.

Brown fat. Also known as "brown adipose tissue" (BAT). This type of fat contains many mitochondria that burn fat to create heat and energy.

Cardiorespiratory fitness. How your heart and lungs work together to establish overall fitness. Cardiorespiratory fitness is achieved by moving large muscle groups for extended periods of time. This type of fitness is a primary predictor of cardiovascular events and death.

Circadian rhythm. The internal 24-hour clock that regulates hormone release, body temperature, sleep, and other biological functions. Circadian rhythms are physical, mental and behavioral changes responding primarily to light and darkness in an organism's environment. They are found in most living things, including animals, plants, and many tiny microbes.

Cytokines. Inflammatory chemicals produced by visceral fat. Cytokines are linked to insulin resistance, heart disease, and other health problems.

Dopamine. A neurotransmitter (brain chemical) that helps regulate the body's reward and motivation system. Dopamine makes us feel good and motivates us toward action. In the obese, the dopamine response system is dampened. The result is that the obese tend to have to eat more than their normal weight counterparts to get the same kind of pleasurable response.

Dumping syndrome. A side effect of eating too many carbohydrates when you have a gastric bypass. Symptoms of dumping syndrome last about 30–45 minutes and include sweating, flushed skin, rapid heart rate, hypotension, nausea, diarrhea, and shakiness.

Duodenum. The first section of the intestine that comes after the stomach. In a normal digestive tract, nutrients enter the duodenum and the nearby pancreas senses any sugars and carbohydrates and secretes insulin.

Free fatty acids (FFAs). Also known as non-esterified fatty acids (NEFA). Free fatty acids are derived from triglycerides. These are important sources of energy in moderate amounts, but high levels of FFAs cause insulin resistance and heart disease.

Gastric bypass. Also known as *Roux-en-Y procedure.* This bariatric surgery involves creating a small stomach pouch that attaches directly to the intestines, bypassing both the stomach and the *duodenum.*

GERD. Gastroesophageal reflux disease (GERD) is a chronic digestive disease. GERD occurs when stomach acid or, occasionally, stomach content, flows back into your food pipe (esophagus). The backwash (reflux) irritates the lining of your esophagus and causes GERD.

Ghrelin. A hormone produced by the stomach that regulates hunger. Ghrelin also slows the metabolism to burn energy and body fat more slowly.

Gut hormones. A term used to describe hormones secreted by the stomach, pancreas, and intestines that control various digestive functions. Known gut hormones include *ghrelin* and *neuropeptide Y*, among others.

Hypothalamus. The part of the brain that is involved with hunger, metabolism, body temperature, and hormone production.

Insulin. A hormone secreted by the pancreas that allows cells in the body to use blood glucose (or sugar) for energy.

Insulin resistance. A condition where the cells in the body are unable to use the hormone insulin to "unlock" the cells and process glucose for energy. People with type 2 diabetes are usually insulin resistant.

Lap-Band®. See *Adjustable gastric banding.*

Leptin. A hormone produced by the fat cells. Leptin helps regulate satiety by sending an "all full" signal to the brain to reduce hunger and increase energy expenditure.

Malabsorptive procedure. A bariatric surgery procedure that changes the way the digestive tract works and how nutrients are absorbed. *Gastric bypass* is a malabsorptive procedure.

Melatonin. A hormone secreted by the pineal gland that helps regulate sleep.

Metabolic syndrome. A group of five health-related traits that raises the risk of heart disease, diabetes, and stroke. The five risk factors are large waist circumference, high triglycerides, low HDL cholesterol, high blood pressure, and high fasting blood sugar levels.

Metabolism. The biological processes and chemical changes within the body by which we burn caloric energy to power bodily functions.

Mindless eating. Also called distracted eating, this term is used to describe the act of eating without paying attention to the food. People often engage in mindless eating when they snack or have a meal in front of the television. Mindless eating can cause overeating.

Monogenic obesity. A rare form of obesity caused by a genetic mutation.

Neuropeptide Y. This brain chemical stimulates hunger and weight gain. It may also trigger a preference for a high-carbohydrate diet.

Obstructive sleep apnea. A sleep disorder that occurs when the throat muscles relax and block the airway, causing disruption to breathing and snoring. People who are over-weight and obese are at risk for this condition.

Polycystic ovary syndrome. Polycystic ovary syndrome (PCOS) is a common endocrine system disorder among women of reproductive age. Women with PCOS may have enlarged ovaries that contain small collections of fluid—called follicles—located in each ovary as seen during an ultrasound exam. Infrequent or prolonged menstrual periods, excess hair growth, acne, and obesity can all occur in women with polycystic ovary syndrome.

Premorbidity. Proceeding or happening before the onset of a disease or health condition. For example, prediabetes is a premorbid state to type 2 diabetes.

Pseudotumor cerebri. A condition in which the pressure inside the skull is increased. The brain is affected in a way that the condition appears to be—but is not—a tumor.

Resting metabolic rate (RMR). The amount of energy we expend as human beings when we are at rest. It represents the energy required to maintain vital bodily functions such as breathing, heart rate, and blood pressure.

Restrictive procedure. A *bariatric surgery* procedure that restricts the size of the stomach (or makes it smaller). *Sleeve gastrectomy* is a restrictive procedure.

Roux-en-Y procedure. See *Gastric bypass.*

Satiety. A feeling of fullness. Many overweight and obese people have disruptions in the hormones and bodily processes that govern satiety signals.

Sleeve gastrectomy. This restrictive bariatric surgery involves amputating 80 percent of the stomach.

Subcutaneous fat. Fat that is just under the skin.

Total energy expenditure (TEE). The amount of energy we use up on all bodily functions and activity.

Triglyceride. Triglycerides are a type of fat. Your body makes some and other triglycerides come from the food you eat. Extra calories are turned into triglycerides and stored in fat cells for later use. If you eat more calories than your body needs, your triglyceride level may be high.

Venous stasis disease. Venous insufficiency is a problem with the flow of blood from the veins of the legs back to the heart. It's also called chronic venous insufficiency or chronic venous stasis.

Visceral fat. The fat that surrounds our organs and can collect around the waistline. Excess visceral fat generates *cytokines* that can cause *insulin resistance*, heart disease, and other health problems.

Waist circumference. A measure of abdominal (visceral) fat. Women should have less than 35 inches and men should have less than 40 inches to reduce cardiometabolic health risk.

Weight bias. Also known as weight stigma. Obese and overweight people may be perceived as lacking willpower instead of others recognizing that they have a chronic health condition. They may also experience discrimination due to their weight.

Weight plateau. A leveling off of weight loss. Weight plateaus often occur when the body adjusts to caloric restriction by lowering the metabolic rate.

White fat. Most of the fat tissue in adults is white fat or white adipose tissue (WAT). This type of fat does not contain the numerous mitochondria found in *brown fat* and *beige fat.*

Zeitgeber. An environmental cue that helps synchronize our circadian clock, such as light.

Index

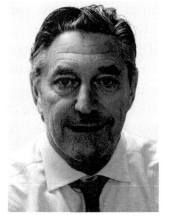 **Steven Lamm**, MD, is a practicing internist, faculty member at New York University School of Medicine, and the Director of the NYU Preston Robert Tisch Center for Men's Health. He is the author/co-author of several popular health and wellness books, including *Redefining Prostate Cancer* (Spry, 2013).

Dr. Lamm regularly offers his expertise on a wide variety of health- and medical-related topics. He has appeared on *The Oprah Winfrey Show, Today, Nightline, Dateline, Fox News, The View*, and the BBC.

A graduate of Columbia University and New York University School of Medicine, Dr. Lamm is the recipient of numerous honors, including American Bariatric Society Recognition Award, Alpha Omega Alpha Award, and New York Founders Day Award. Dr. Lamm is active in clinical research and is a panel physician for the New York State Athletic Commission.

George Alexander Fielding

George Alexander Fielding, MD, FRACS, FRCS (Eng), FRCS (Glas), Professor of Surgery at NYU School of Medicine, is a pioneer in laparoscopic and bariatric surgery. Dr. Fielding studied medicine at the University of Queensland, graduating in 1979, and completed his medical training at the Royal Brisbane Hospital. During his postgraduate training, he developed interests in laparoscopic and hepato-biliary-pancreatic surgery and then pursued advanced training in the field in Britain and Switzerland. In 1989, he returned to Royal Brisbane Hospital as a staff surgeon and then later founded the Wesley Obesity Clinic at the Wesley Hospital, also in Brisbane, earning a reputation for his expertise in laparoscopic, bariatric, and hepato-biliary surgery. To date, he has performed more than 8,000 bariatric surgeries. Dr. Fielding's expertise also lies in laparoscopic abdominal hernias, particularly complex paraesophageal and abdominal wall hernias.

Dr. Fielding has been instrumental in the development of laparoscopic surgery and has taught the techniques to surgeons around the world and has published more than 150 journal articles, abstracts, and book chapters.

He is a Fellow of the Royal Australasian College of Surgeons and the Royal College of Surgeons (England). In addition, he is a member of the American Society of Metabolic and Bariatric Surgery, the Society of American Gastrointestinal and Endoscopic Surgeons, and New York Surgical Society.

Dr. Fielding underwent Lap-Band® surgery himself in 1999, giving him an unusually personal perspective on this special group of patients. He was named a Castle Connolly Top Doctor in 2011, 2012, and 2013.

Christine Ren-Fielding

Christine Ren-Fielding, MD, FACS, FASMBS, Professor of Surgery at NYU School of Medicine, is considered by many to be the leading Lap-Band® Surgeon in the United States. She has performed more than 4,000 gastric band procedures.

Dr. Ren-Fielding obtained her medical degree at Tufts University School of Medicine in Boston, followed by a residency in surgery at NYU Medical Center. Dr. Ren-Fielding went on to complete a fellowship in advanced laparoscopic surgery at Mount Sinai Medical Center, where she was involved as faculty in the minimally invasive bariatric surgery workshops to train surgeons in laparoscopic bariatric surgery. Dr. Ren-Fielding founded and is the director of the NYU Langone Weight Management Program and is the Chief of the Division of Bariatric

Surgery. She has been involved extensively in research in vascular medicine, angiogenesis, and bariatric surgery; she has authored more than 35 scientific articles and five book chapters and has lectured worldwide.

Dr. Ren-Fielding was instrumental in spearheading the creation of 11 new CPT codes for bariatric surgery. This has enabled insurance companies to cover these operations, which previously denied millions of Americans insurance coverage for these life-saving operations.

Dr. Ren-Fielding is recognized nationally and internationally for her contributions to the field of bariatric surgery. She is the recipient of a 2004 YWCA Woman's Achievement Award, has appeared on *Oprah*, was profiled in Crain's 2005 special issue on New York's Rising Stars, and has been a Castle Connolly Top Doctor since 2005.

Norman Sussman

Norman Sussman, MD, is Professor of Psychiatry at the New York University School of Medicine and also Director of the Treatment Resistant Depression Program and Medical Director of the Steven and Alexandra Cohen Military Family Clinic at the NYU Langone Medical Center. Dr. Sussman most recently served as Interim Chair of the Department of Psychiatry and as Associate Dean for Continuing Medical Education at the medical school.

A graduate of Queens College in New York, Dr. Sussman obtained a Master of Public Administration degree from the Robert F. Wagner Graduate School of Public Service, where he majored in health care administration. He received his M.D. from New York Medical College and completed his residency in psychiatry at Metropolitan Hospital and Westchester County Medical Center. He joined the faculty at NYU School of Medicine in 1980 and served both as director of inpatient psychiatry at Tisch Hospital and director of residency training in psychiatry. Dr. Sussman has been active in medical education for his entire career and developed one of the first university-based review courses in general psychiatry and in psychopharmacology. He is committed to the continuing education of both psychiatric and non-psychiatric physicians in the rapidly changing field of psychopharmacology.

Dr. Sussman served on the American Psychiatric Association's Task Force for the development of the American Psychiatric Association's *Diagnostic and Statistical Manual of Mental Disorders, 3rd edition* (DSM-III) and helped develop the criteria for Factitious and Somatoform Disorders. He is a Distinguished Fellow of the American Psychiatric Association, and he received that organization's Certificate of Recognition for Excellence in Medical Student Education. Dr. Sussman has been an investigator for numerous clinical trials involving treatment for anxiety and mood disorders. He writes and lectures extensively on psychopharmacology both in this country and around the world, and has a private practice in Manhattan.

Dr. Sussman is a regular contributor to medical literature. He is a contributing editor for the Biological Therapies section in Kaplan & Sadock's *Comprehensive Textbook of Psychiatry*, and a co-author of *The Handbook of Psychiatric Drug Therapy*.